治癌实录 2

中晚期癌症·名家手记

吴锦 著

中国科学技术出版社
·北京·

图书在版编目（CIP）数据

治癌实录 2，中晚期癌症·名家手记 / 吴锦著 . —北京：中国科学技术出版社，2017.9（2021.4 重印）

ISBN 978-7-5046-7650-4

Ⅰ . ①治… Ⅱ . ①吴… Ⅲ . ①癌－中西医结合－诊疗 Ⅳ . ① R73

中国版本图书馆 CIP 数据核字（2017）第 206676 号

策划编辑	焦健姿
责任编辑	黄维佳
装帧设计	长天印艺
责任校对	马思志
责任印制	马宇晨

出　　版	中国科学技术出版社
发　　行	中国科学技术出版社有限公司发行部
地　　址	北京市海淀区中关村南大街 16 号
邮　　编	100081
发行电话	010-62173865
传　　真	010-62179148
网　　址	http://www.cspbooks.com.cn

开　　本	850mm×1168mm　1/32
字　　数	118 千字
印　　张	6.5
版　　次	2017 年 9 月第 1 版
印　　次	2021 年 4 月第 2 次印刷
印　　刷	天津翔远印刷有限公司
书　　号	ISBN 978-7-5046-7650-4 / R · 2071
定　　价	28.00 元

（凡购买本社图书，如有缺页、倒页、脱页者，本社发行部负责调换）

修善第一 旨在救人

吴锦教授留念

陈可冀

壬辰端午前

▲中国科学院院士陈可冀教授题词

内容提要

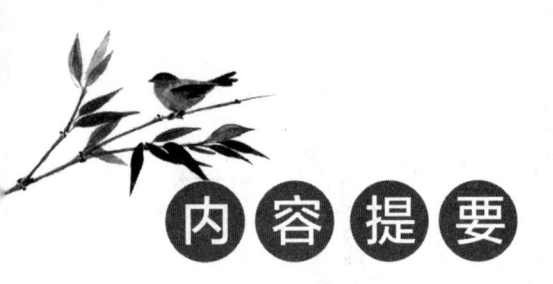

本书作者为资深中医药治疗癌症专家，她将自己从事中医药抗癌工作的亲身经历与智慧融会到书中，介绍了作者对癌症预防、治疗等方面的看法，以及有关防癌、治癌的基本知识，然后以深入浅出、通俗易懂的写作手法，对生命修复抗癌中医药治疗癌症的原则及方法做了全面论述，并附有大量真实病案。本书所述病案均基于客观事实，没有任何夸大，希望对广大中西医工作者、癌症患者及其家人有所帮助。

前言

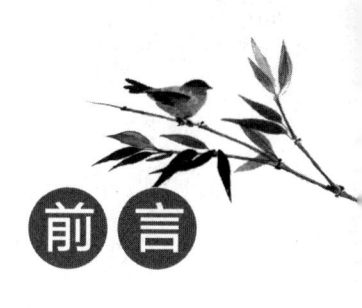

癌症是全球最严重的疾病之一，其发病率越来越高，死亡数字更是年年攀升。当前现代医学对付癌症，主要靠化疗、放疗及手术治疗，患者往往竭力忍受治疗所带来的痛苦，在治疗过程中离世，或是因癌症复发、癌细胞转移、器官衰竭而死亡。这些例子多不胜数，许多人认为癌症等于绝症。本人通过生命修复疗法，应用中医药治疗癌症取得了良好效果。所以说癌症并不是绝症，癌症也不等于死亡，关键在于治疗方法上必须革新和转变，在医学理论上也必须发展和创新。

为了鼓励癌症患者本人及其家人，我将近年来通过生命修复抗癌中医药治疗的经验和体会编撰成书，以期鼓励更多患者与癌症抗争而非放弃。书中所有病案都基于客观事实，没有任何夸大，并尽量展示出治疗前后客观的检测报告，以确认其真实性。因治癌是一个非常复杂的过程，必须深刻洞悉患者的身体、疾病、原因、治疗过程中的变化，以及相应的治疗方案与方药的变化等，所以不可能用一个或几个药方解决全部问题。那些用一个家传秘方或什么奇效偏方就治好了癌症的说法，更是无稽之谈。此外，临床上好转，肿瘤稳定或消失之后，还需要更重要的措施和治疗，以防止复发、转移等。本人诚惶诚恐，生怕误导患者。

本书的宗旨在于：①提出癌症预防的重要性；②鼓励患者，增强患者及其家人抗癌的信心和勇气；③对同行们抛砖引玉。个人的观点不一定都对，希望多多批评指导，并希望有更好的方法不断问世。

本人对现代医学的生理、病理、药理实验、临床等方面都进行过多年的研究工作，但在现实治疗癌症工作中，感到中医药更具有优势。许多大病、重病，包括癌症，并不能用当前高科技、现代化的先进手段获得良好效果。在攻克癌症的

前言

多年研究中，本人不得不另辟新途，寻找更好、更有效、更切合实际的方法，这就是生命修复抗癌中医药治疗。大量病案说明中医药能够治癌。

医学本身并不需要以中医、西医区分，两者都是人类治疗疾病、战胜疾病和向前发展的财富。西医和中医的发展都没有完结，都需要不断加深认识、重新认识、继续探求、继续研究。

感谢我的导师，中国科学院资深院士陈可冀教授为本书题词。本人会在攻克癌症的领域中继续努力和研究，为中医药治癌尽个人微薄之力，同时，期望得到更多的支持。

吴　锦

目录

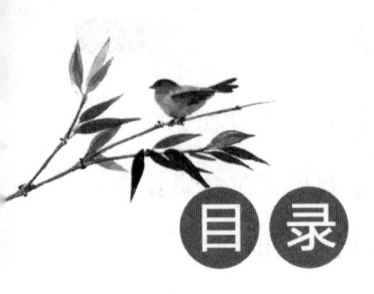

上篇 抗癌养生篇

癌症的预防 …………………………………… 2

看似无关却有关 ……………………………… 5

重视饮食 ……………………………………… 10

无毒无害养生治癌 …………………………… 19

另辟新途癌症可治 …………………………… 22

对抗癌症疼痛 ………………………………… 25

患者消瘦要调理 ……………………………… 28

夫妻癌现象 …………………………………… 31

审证求因治疗癌性胸腹水 …………………… 33

抗癌治疗与带瘤生存 ………………………… 35

癌症复发和转移勿放弃 ……………………… 37

中医药治癌新观念 …………………………… 39

带病延年养生长寿 …………………………… 42

下篇　抗癌治验录

抗癌明星，百岁寿星 …………………… 46

晚期鼻咽癌康复 ………………………… 49

降服肺癌脑转移 ………………………… 58

没做化疗和放疗 ………………………… 66

把握阴阳调平衡，肺癌已度十八年 …… 69

治九旬长者食管癌 ……………………… 78

补中消瘤，转危为安 …………………… 85

无毒无害治大病 ………………………… 95

命余一至三个月，补正祛邪续新篇 …… 103

肝癌劫后获新生 ………………………… 110

战胜肝癌，喜获麟儿 …………………… 116

消瘤扶正，正常生活 …………………… 124

抗乳癌加保胎，母子平安 ……………… 130

晚期子宫癌康复 ………………………… 138

末期子宫颈癌，重拾生命年华 ………… 144

坚持攻坚补正，战胜晚期转移癌 ……… 148

晚期肾癌骨转移，治疗四个月可爬山 … 154

晚期癌症创奇迹，勇征喜马拉雅山 ……… 162

两种恶癌集一身，抗癌疗法显奇功 ……… 171

击退癌魔，笔端生辉 ……… 176

攻坚通络，消散大量肿瘤兼腹水 ……… 184

停化疗扶阳祛毒，晚期肿瘤全消失 ……… 188

咳嗽原从腮腺来，清热解毒助瘤消 ……… 197

编者按

　　本书所述病案均采用专业的抗癌中医药治疗，如有患者欲尝试中医药治疗，应求治于有丰富肿瘤专科经验并专长于抗癌中医药治疗且具有信誉的专业注册中医师。

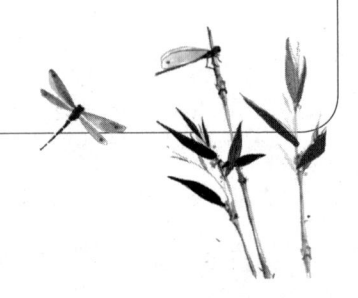

上篇

抗癌养生篇

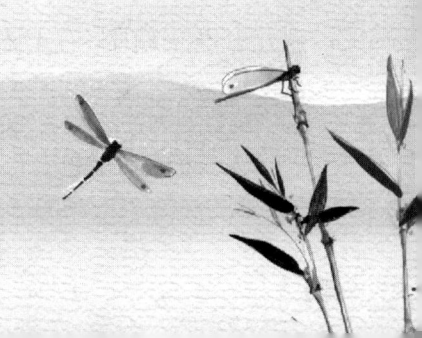

癌症的预防

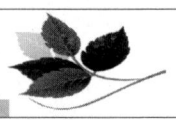

注重癌症的预防

尽管现代医学不断发展,癌症的发病率和死亡率却越来越高。常听人说,在我们这代人中,癌症以前是一种很少见的严重疾病;其后逐渐有越来越多的人患上癌症;再过数年后,就经常得知身旁的亲戚朋友、公司的同事、甚至自己的家人罹患癌症;再过些时日,恐怕癌症"就找上了自己"。

统计显示,近三十年来,癌症的发病率直线飙升,2006年中国的肺癌发病率是1973年的465%。2007年全球死于癌症的人数是760万,就是说,每天有两万多人死于癌症。专家预计,到2020年,全球每年死于癌症的人数将达到1500万。美国国家疾病控制中心(CDC)预测,如果未来美国人的平均寿命能到九十岁,美国将有47%的男性公民和32%的女性公民死于癌症。

人人都有可能患上癌症,这是大家不愿又不得不承认的事实。癌症的预防，已经成为非常重要、非常急迫的问题。

怎样预防癌症呢？人们感到茫然。不少医生、专家也感到茫然。如果对某种疾病的发病原因、发展过程心中无数，如何谈论预防呢？

常听说癌症患者化疗到生命最后一分钟。有的患者经过漫长的化疗，结果无效。那么，医生就会建议选择另一种化疗药，再试，又无效，再重新换一种化疗药，再试试，直到患者不能再试了为止。这样的治疗，一直都存在，又如何谈到癌症的预防呢？

我们认为，癌症是可以预防的，而且癌症的预防非常重要且刻不容缓。癌症的发生有相当多已知原因，我们应针对这些原因积极采取预防措施。

导致癌症的原因

1. 饮食因素

饮食结构不正确，包括进食不洁食物、霉变食物、不当加工的食物、腌制食物、大量不当的肉类食品、刺激性食物、食物的防腐剂、不当的添加剂、合成色素等。当今的食物中，采用的添加剂真是五花八门，像膨松剂、增香剂、嫩肉精、瘦肉精、增鲜剂、增稠剂、催熟剂、保鲜剂等，数不胜数。如果长期大量进食这样的食物，会增加患癌的机会。

2. 不良行为

如长期抽烟酗酒、不良卫生习惯、不洁或不当的性生活等。

3. 环境污染

如汽车废气、工业污染、化工厂烟雾、放射性环境污染（如日本的核污染）等。

4. 理化致癌因素

接触有毒害的理化因素，滥用药物，特别是长期不合理地使用化学合成药物，如性激素、各类激素、抗排异药物、解热镇痛药物、抗癌药、止痛药、抗生素等。

5. 精神因素

长期存在压抑、紧张、悲伤、痛苦、愤怒、嫉恨等不良情绪会增加患癌的风险。

6. 遗传因素

家族中有癌症患者，也会增加其他人的患癌风险。

看似无关却有关

维护生态平衡

当今高科技的发展,给大自然造成了许多破坏。河水断流、地震山崩都不时地发生着。人类在红尘中日渐迷失本性,沉浸在物欲横流的喧嚣世界。然而我们人类和这个世界上所有还存在的一切生物一样,都是大自然的生命,都是物竞天择的产物。恐龙灭绝了,但还有无数的生物因为不能生存而灭绝了或濒临灭绝。希望人类不要跟在这些物种后面重蹈覆辙!

当今人们做了大量破坏自然规律、违背生态平衡的事,例如大量破坏森林资源,大量捕杀濒危动物,大量杀生。人们追求物欲、性感,却忽视了金钱买不到的东西,例如良好的道德,例如阳光、空气、雨露、水源等。

遵循自然规律

从各种古籍的记载中可以看到,古时候也是有癌症的,例如翻花、症瘕、乳岩、阴疽……等都是有关恶性肿瘤的描述。但是，那时癌症绝对没有这么普遍，所以并无大量这种疾病的专著。在近代，物质生活比较困乏的年代，癌症也不是十分常见，而随着生活的现代化和科技的发展，癌症也在迅速地发展着。

数千年前，我们的祖先就知道，大自然是有规律可循的。我们要顺应大自然的规律，而不是处处违逆、破坏大自然的规律。所以不要追求时髦，而应崇尚自然的生活。如果人人都将自己置身于大自然的怀抱，则会减少许多疾病和烦恼。

大雁随候而迁，熊蛇入冬则眠。顺应自然，万物繁华，抗逆自然，必遭天谴，这就是生命的规则。

一年有春、夏、秋、冬四季的变化，人体的生理功能，也是跟随着这种变化，体现出阴阳互根、阴阳消长的基本规律，保持生生不息和健康。春升、夏浮、秋降、冬藏，是天地气机的升降规律，在人体也一样有这种气机和变化的规律。如果不去遵循，就会导致各种生理功能逆乱。轻微时现代化的仪器查不出，查出时已是大病。春暖、夏热、秋凉、冬寒，是人们应该去经历的。四季如春的生活，是时尚，而不一定合理。不是说不要使用冷气机和暖气机，而是在一定范围内，人体应该经受到春天温暖、气温适宜，夏天炎热、腠理汗出，秋天凉燥、毛孔关闭，冬天寒冷、气血收藏的正常自然过程，人体的气机才会有正常升降循回，才符合自然规律，才不易因气血逆乱、气血障碍而生病。

人的生命与大自然是息息相关的，上文只是举例说明了人与自然的关系，中国古时的先哲们正是因为看到并认识到这种规律，才提出天人合一的观点并逐步发展了中医药学。

而西方医学的先哲们则看到了细菌对人体的伤害，发明了抗生素，这两种完全不同的哲理和思路，都值得尊重。

曾几何时，只有过年才能吃到的山珍海味、大鱼大肉，现在天天都在吃，甚至一顿餐不吃都不行。反季节的食物越来越多，不在其季节生长而收获，看似相同，食之无味。还有为了增加牛奶的产量，而给奶牛使用大量激素……这些现象到底是文明的进步还是倒退；对健康有益还是有害都值得我们认真沉思。

观念回归

许多事物有利也有弊，经济越进步，社会越现代化，难治的病也越多。因此不妨将有些观念，回归到旧时、穷时、古时，寻找解决的办法。

1. 顺天应时，作息有序

大自然中日出月归、潮涨汐落，都有着特定的规律，人们应该遵循这个时间的规律而不是有意去破坏和对抗。古人早有日出而作、日落而息的说法，便是顺应天地的自然做法。现代人常通宵熬夜，整晚不眠，大白天太阳出来了，却又昏睡整日。这对于事业的发展或许是很有用的，但长期下去，对身体的生理功能，一定有不好的影响。

2. 生活安稳

当今外面的世界很精彩，声色、喧嚣、旅途，虽然生活丰富多样，但对人体气血的涵养，却远不如安静、稳定的生活。

3. 心境平和

社会竞争激烈，争斗冲突不断，也许是社会发展的需要，却不是维护健康的需要。保持平和的心态，用愉快的心情来度过每日平凡的时光；不斤斤计较，不争强好胜，淡泊名利，超脱世俗，将荣华当作过眼云烟，视苦难为人之常情；常施援手，乐于助人……如果有修养，就去追求这高尚的精神境界；如果无修养，就设法做到与世无争，也能排解大量的烦恼。

4. 劳逸适度，因人而异

流水不腐、户枢不蠹，流动的水不会发臭；经常转动的门轴不会腐烂，比喻经常运动的东西不易受到侵蚀。人们以此引伸到要经常运动,才能保持健康,这原本是无可非议的。但如果运用不当也会出现很多问题。比如有的患者身体已很虚弱,仍不惜每日拖着疲惫不堪的身躯去跑步、爬山,做自己的体力难以承受的运动,以为这样就可以治好疾病,结果却是更加虚弱,事与愿违。在这种情况下,调理生命的阴阳平衡更为重要。晚期癌症患者,在力所能及的情况下做一些缓慢的运动,如太极拳等则更为合适。

重视饮食

怎样吃才有益于健康？怎样吃才有利于疾病尽早康复？这是大多数患者和家人都会问到的问题。

对于怎样吃才健康的问题，以往的许多宣传、报道甚至深入人心的饮食法，都是有错误的。人们必须改变许多饮食观念，例如有的患者一日进食五至六餐；有的患者一日要喝几次高浓度的葡萄糖水；有的患者大量地服用维生素药片；有的患者止痛西药当饭吃，即使很久不痛了也一定准时服用；还有的有点感冒头痛，就尽快服用抗生素……问他们为什么这样？他们都会认真地说，为了尽早治好疾病，为了尽快恢复健康。但是这些做法是错误的，应该尽快纠正。

拒绝过多美味

饮食中不要追求美味佳肴，对许多人来讲，这是困难且不可思议的。重点是要有观念的改变。所谓美味，不外乎山珍海味、大鱼大肉，如果没有大量的食品添加剂，是不会有现代的美味食物的。更有许多商人，为追求利润而刻意生产口感特别、色泽鲜艳的食品，却不顾吃进去的后果。此类食品，少量进食不一定能表现出明显的症状。但长期、大量地进食后可能导致多种疾病。人们也许想不到，这些疾病与他们的饮食习惯有关。

《黄帝内经》中早就指出，"膏粱之变，足生大丁"，膏粱是厚味，泛指煎炒炙爆的高脂肪食物。足是能够，足够之意。大丁，泛指疮疡肿毒及突出于某部分的痈疽，也即当代所指的肿瘤之类。意思就是说，吃许多美味、油腻的食物，能够生出这一类的疾病。从现在的烹制手段来看，如果食物没有色、香、味的过分加工，怎么会产生美味呢？而这些加工过程，又怎样能够没有大量的食品添加剂呢？

拒绝高动物蛋白、高营养

不要吃得太好，少肉食、不要高营养的饮食原则。例如，获美国癌症研究终身成就奖的 Colin Campbell 曾指出，动物性膳食及牛奶会增加许多癌症的发病率。世界癌症研究基金会等权威组织，曾于 2007 年在全球多个城市发布过《肿瘤饮食与指南》，探讨分析了世界各地数万份调查报告及研究结果，得出一个结论，即红肉可导致直肠癌等癌症的发生。

有些癌症患者吃各种高营养物质，特别是这几年，吃营养粉与蛋白粉成为时尚,但没多久,这些人中有一些出现了肿瘤复发、淋巴结增大、肿瘤扩散的情况。有位患者,李太,五十多岁,她是位营养师,非常重视各种营养的补充。当她得知自己患上淋巴癌后,除了补充大量动物蛋白,更每日饮用两大杯营养蛋白粉。结果肿瘤迅速增大,体质急速恶化,她吃的营养越多,人反而越瘦。虽然积极接受化疗,但也无法挽救生命。这样的沉痛教训有很多,我们应当有所认识。高营养、高动物蛋白,不一定带来健康,对于癌症患者更是如此。

很多中药和植物药都有改善体质的作用。合理的中药和合理的膳食结构可以增强体质和免疫力,关键是要因人而异,辨证施治,辨证择食。

许多人以为,动物蛋白比植物蛋白好。这也是不确定的。

德国 MAXPLANCK 中心营养研究得出的结论是,植物蛋白优于动物蛋白,特别是绿色植物,含有多种优质的蛋白质。其他如坚果类、菜类及黄豆等都含有氨基酸蛋白质,这些优点不亚于动物蛋白,结论是植物类食物应是最好的食物来源。而且植物类食物还含有丰富的多种微量元素和许多抗癌元素。

有权威性的研究机构指出,长期大量饮用牛奶会有坏处。因为其中的雌激素等其他激素,都是奶类中致癌的物质。有外国肿瘤专家认为,除了发展中国家的儿童和营养不良的成人,不建议一般人喝太多牛奶。

素食为主

大量食肉或以肉食为主的坏处，是容易看到且容易理解的。有些有毒物质，并不一定能够用当今的检测技术检验出来，但是用现代的医学知识分析，以下几点是可以肯定的：

（1）动物在现代的饲养过程中，完全脱离正常的生长环境，被迫生长在窄小恶劣的人工环境中，这使得动物为适宜生存从初生时，机体就开始分泌各种不正常的有害物质来对抗这种非自然的生活。

（2）为降低死亡，缩短养殖过程，动物会被强迫进食或注射各种药物，例如抗生素、生长激素、镇静剂、瘦肉精、多肉精等，这些物质会大量残留于动物体内成为毒素。

（3）动物吃进的各种不洁的、有害的物质。

（4）动物体内本身的疾病、肿瘤及生长环境中的寄生虫、细菌、病毒等并不是全部都能检测出来，或者并不是全部要求检测出来。

（5）动物在被宰杀过程中，由于"应激"反应，痛苦、挣扎、愤怒、绝望、抗拒而分泌出各种毒素。

（6）动物死亡后，自身分解而产生各种毒素。

（7）肉类在制作过程中，加入了各种防腐剂、添加剂、矫味剂等有害物质。

（8）违反正常生理过程的人为制造的肉食，例如给予特殊饲料喂饲食动物，然后以此制成的小牛肉、乳猪肉等等。大量的动物脂肪、动物蛋白、内分泌激素等会对人体产生危害。

再如饲养过程中使用大量的激素，导致现代的乳牛从两岁就开始分泌乳汁。研究经发现，这种牛奶中的激素会诱发卵巢癌细胞繁殖，加速癌细胞生长。

饮食有节

饮食过量，有害无益。尽量吃饱是错误的饮食观念，这样会使胃肠负担过重，全身气血壅塞。而少食才会使人体气血处于生机勃勃的状态。

《黄帝内经》中就指出"饮食自倍，脾胃乃伤"。南朝齐梁时期，著名医药学家陶弘景在《养生延年录》中也说过："所食愈少、心愈开、年愈寿，所食愈多、心愈塞、年愈损焉"。可见古人早已知道饮食有节的重要性。

国内外许多研究也表明，经常饮食过度，不仅会使消化系统长期负担过重，也会导致免疫功能下降，大脑早衰。摄入的过多的热量会引起许多"富贵病"和"现代文明病"，例如肥胖症、高血压、糖尿病、高血脂、动脉硬化等，许多病与癌症也有一定关系。

饮食清淡、粗茶淡饭，才是使人长寿健康的饮食观念，也只有这样，才能避免吃进去过多的毒素，并且有效避免多种疾病，使人体气血运行更加畅通无阻。

慎重入口

许多化学合成物品入口之前要小心谨慎。如抗生素，就是典型例证。

抗生素对人有毒副作用，这是众所周知的事，如使用不当会对肝肾功能、脑神经及听觉神经造成损害。因此，年老体弱之人和儿童使用抗生素更应特别慎重。

抗生素会使病菌产生耐药性，若盲目使用新的、更高级的抗生素，患者体内的病菌继而又对新的抗生素产生耐药性，一旦再发生感染，那就无药可医。

抗生素还可能加重病情或造成二重感染。例如肠道菌群失调就是抗生素影响正常细菌的生长及繁殖，破坏了肠道生态，影响肠道正常功能的结果。

抗生素也可能延误病情。有些病本不适合用抗生素治疗，结果因滥用抗生素，破坏了体内的菌群的平衡，产生了新的疾病。

举个例子：有一个男孩子的年龄只有四岁，但有近两年的时间经常发热，通常每星期都有三至五天发热。初时家人与医生都以为是感冒引起，每次到医院求医，医生都会开退热药和抗生素。随着服用这些药物的时间增多，体温不退反高，甚至39℃以上，超过40℃的次数也越来越多。而小男孩在长期服食抗生素后，出现了极大的不良反应，脸色青黄、食欲缺乏及身体消瘦。服用太多退热药及抗生素严重影响了他的身体发育，使他瘦小虚弱，而发热却总是不退。父母和家人伤透了脑筋，医生也用尽了新型、高效的抗生素，最后宣布无药可医，因此男孩的长辈把他带来用中医药治疗。

孩子很小而中药很苦，针灸治疗很痛，但父母仍决心孤注一掷，再麻烦、再心痛也要试试。因为这样小的孩子，这样继续高热下去，父母、长辈和孩子本人都难以承受。孩子虽然哭闹，却十分听话懂事。他知道虽然很痛很苦，但都是为了给他治病。就这样，在孩子的哭闹和坚持中陆续治疗了几个月，高热逐渐降为低热，发热的次数逐渐减少，以后慢慢恢复到了健康状态。

还有许多方面，如养殖业，因经济成本而滥用化学药物和抗生素。许多鸡、鸭、猪等养殖场，在动物饲料中掺杂抗生素，借此预防一些动物疾病。抗生素存在动物体内，人类食用后便转移到人体。

水果蔬菜等农作物亦有使用不同的化学合成药、抗生素的现象,这些物质残留在植物上,污染了食物源头,同样对人体构成危害。

少去餐馆

当今的餐馆,是会友、社交的场所之一。人们常去餐馆,甚至每日都在餐馆,不免带来相当多的问题。例如追求美味,暴饮暴食,进食大量含调味剂等的食品,各种烟酒、味精、鸡精越多越好,烹饪油反复加热,不合理的烹调过程,食品的储存方式等,都会对身体产生一定的影响。

天然最佳

天然食物,指没有经过化学加工、商品过程、制成品处理的食物。

以最流行的各种饮料来讲,有些人不喝水,每天只喝饮料,以为多喝饮料身体便好,这种想法其实非常错误。饮料中含有多种不同的、非天然的物质,以增加色、香、味与口感,但口感好并不是有利健康的标志。碳酸饮料中,含过量的二氧化碳、碳酸,会影响人体的消化功能,造成胃肠道功能障碍。尤其是可乐还含有磷酸,长期饮用会使大量的磷酸渗入,可造成钙稀疏、钙磷比例失调，造成骨骼发育缓慢、骨质疏松。

因人而异，辨证择食

无论是养生，还是治病，都应该有整体观念和辨证思想。有些医生治病时，如果因为所患的是同一种病，例如都是肝癌或肺炎，所给的药物和治疗都是一样的，这显然不对。如果只看到某个器官生病、发炎、长瘤，而不顾及局部组织与全身整体的相互关系和影响，也是只见树木、不见森林的做法。

辨证择食，就是了解食物的性味及功用，又考虑到个人身体素质、性别、年龄、疾病变化等各个方面，而有针对性地选择饮食。

虽然许多食物的性味和功效没有药物那么强烈，但是通过经常及多次地进食，也能起到一定的调理和协助治疗的作用。当然，如果吃的食物正好与个体所需药性相反，就对疾病的治疗产生相反的作用。

例如阳虚体质适宜吃温热温补的食物，忌吃大寒、生冷的损阳食品；阴虚体质适宜吃滋阴生津的清补食物，忌食生燥、生热的大热上火食物。就是最常见的感冒，也有风寒、风热等不同的辨证分型，感冒时的饮食也对病情的恢复或加重有直接影响。

无毒无害养生治癌

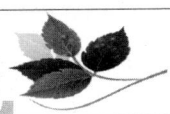

西医治病，是当前社会和医学界的主流。中医治病，在一些城市及地区，仍然是不被重视的。然而，尽管有高科技的现代医疗诊治技术，仍有许多疾病缺乏有效的治疗手段。例如癌症，如果癌症患者在医院已得到了有效的治疗，就不会有患者不得不再来寻求中医药治疗。许多患者已属很晚期，他们由试试看到坚持长期治疗，由不相信到相信和依赖抗癌中医药治疗，说明了中医药治癌思路和措施的正确性。

抗生素的发明，使全球感染性疾病得到了有效的控制。抗生素的使用，挽救了无数的生命。但是使用抗生素杀死细菌的方法，只能治疗细菌感染性的疾病。世上的事情很复杂，各种疾病的发生发展也非常复杂。比如癌症，就不能用一样的战略方式、思维和治疗模式来对待。

到目前为止，虽然美国征服癌症的战争早就宣告失败了，这些征服中曾用的治疗方法，仍然在全球的每个医院中继续使用着。按照这种观念，癌细胞是等同于细菌，是侵入人体的敌人，所以要用战争来消灭它。

要消灭癌症，首先要消灭最大量存在的癌细胞，这就需要做手术切除肿瘤，而且手术的部位和面积要尽可能的大，希望这样可以"根治"。但是，一段时间后，癌细胞又从身体其他部位长出来了，其实并没有根治。

第二，化疗，用各种各样的毒性药物，来毒死所有的癌细胞。但是，正常的细胞也被毒死的不少，而癌细胞无法全部毒死。一种毒药不行，再换一种，或者几种毒药联合化疗，结果是癌细胞照样复发，转移，扩散。

第三，放射治疗（放疗），用放射线烧死癌细胞，面积尽量包括了肿瘤的整个位置，尽管会烧死正常的组织细胞，尽管有严重可怕的后遗症，也要不惜代价将癌细胞烧死。但是一段时间后，癌细胞照样生长出来，或者即使放疗的局部无复发，但肿瘤又在其他部位和器官出现了。

分析这些治疗方法，实际上是和杀死细菌的思路一样的，但癌细胞并不是细菌，所以无法全部杀死，癌症也就不能像是感染性疾病那样容易用抗生素控制。难道不能用另一种思路来考虑问题吗？答案是有的，那就是传统的中医药。在西方医学没有传到东方之前，中医药学是中华民族繁衍昌盛的保护神。在西方医学传入东方之后，传统的中医药曾一度被排斥，冷落，但她从来没有消失。中医药始终在世界上相当大的范围内发挥着治病救人的重要作用。

在西方医学不能有效控制癌症的当今，我们再来更加深入探讨中医药学的治病哲理，进一步研究和发展中医药学的治病机制，探求生命奥秘，是非常有现实意义的，也是非常必要和急需的，后文这些治疗成功的案例，说明运用中医药治疗癌症是走上了正确的征癌之路。

另辟新途癌症可治

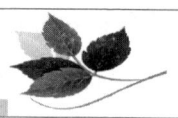

得了癌症不等于死亡。癌症患者经过合理的、有效治疗，是仍然可以带病延年、养生长寿的。然而，要使众多的癌症患者实现这样的理想，仍需要做很多的研究工作和努力。首先，多年来在日常饮食、观念、广告宣传等很多方面都存在误区，而且这些错误观念的影响很大，有些甚至在人们的头脑中根深蒂固。要想有效抗癌，必须要走出诸如治疗要高营养饮食、猛烈杀灭癌细胞、强烈毒性治疗、癌症不可治、只能姑息舒缓等误区。

举个例子：王女士，五十七岁，她被发现患了肠癌后，首先是住院做手术切除了肠及肿瘤，接着是几个月的痛苦治疗。为了不使癌症复发，她坚持做了十二个疗程的化疗，然后又接着做了放疗。但是复查时，却发现肠癌复发，并且转移到了肝。按照医生的要求，她再次住院，再次做手术切除肠的肿瘤及肝脏肿瘤，接着再化疗并加标靶治疗。又经过漫长难熬的治疗后，再次做检查，结果发现肝脏又长出了新的肿瘤，而且比之前更大。

按照主诊医生的说法，这个肿瘤太大又耐药，下一步的治疗，要更换更加强烈的化疗药，来对抗这个更大的肿瘤，待到肿瘤变得小一些时，需要再次做手术来切除肿瘤。王女士就再次接受这种更新更强的化学治疗。但无奈化疗过程中癌指数持续上升，提示化疗效果不好，同时不良反应太大，呕吐、头晕、失眠、脱发等很情况严重。在这种万般无奈的情况下，王女士来接受抗癌中医药治疗。

王女士第一次求诊时，所述说的情况，也许多数医生听后会认为是很正常的、合理的、科学的，但该医师听到后，感到非常吃惊。她说，按照主诊医生的要求，她每日要尽量多地吃肉，只有大量的肉食，才能增加营养、增强体质，配合治疗。即使她胃口很差，经常呕叶，甚至吃肉吃得舌头感到麻木，还是要继续努力不停地大量吃肉。

在接受抗癌中医药治疗后，她首先彻底改变了她的食谱和饮食结构，果断地停止大量肉食，并每日服用中药。王女士并不是十分相信中医药，之前已做了两次手术，正准备做第三次手术，但手术前希望能缩小肿瘤，才来看看。她决定坚持服一段时间中药试试看。

几个月下来她再去检查，希望肿瘤能缩小，而能够有再次做手术的机会。检查结果表明：肝脏的肿瘤已经消失。王女士高兴地说，去医院复诊时，西医也说她不需要再次做手术了。王女士的情况证明，合理的中医药治疗是有效的，及时更正不合理的饮食，用合理的食物配合治疗，也是非常重要的。

对抗癌症疼痛

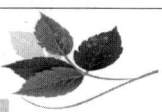

许多癌症患者都有疼痛，有的很严重，有的比较轻微，但多属持久痛症，癌症疼痛的原因大概有以下几种：

（1）肿瘤所造成的疼痛，如肿瘤生长压迫神经、肿瘤造成骨转移、肿瘤增大压迫周围组织、局部膨胀、压力大、循环差等。

（2）治疗过程中造成，如放射线（放疗）所造成的纤维化，组织破坏、化疗所导致的神经病变、手术所造成的组织损伤、手术结扎造成的神经血管损伤等。

（3）与肿瘤相关引起的疼痛，如肿瘤压迫、淋巴水肿、褥疮、与肿瘤相关的关节疼痛等。

常见的镇痛药有口服、舌下含服、皮肤贴片、注射等给药方法。根据疼痛程度不同，给予的止痛药有辅助性止痛药、非鸦片类止痛药和鸦片类止痛药的不同。非鸦片类止痛药常见的不良反应有胃肠道毒性，例如消化不良、胃溃疡、恶心、呕吐、震颤、运动失调、意识混乱、视力障碍、肝肾功能受损、血液系统受损、止痛作用差等。

阿片类镇痛药的不良反应如便秘、恶心、呕吐、昏睡、幻觉、狂躁、呼吸抑制、耐受性、成瘾性、止痛效果不理想等等。

举个例子：张女士，六十三岁，两年前患肠癌，虽经过多次化疗，但于一年前发生骨转移，在多家医院进行治疗，用了大量的吗啡类强止痛药，仍然疼痛剧烈，昼夜难安。无奈之下求助于中医药治疗。经过综合治疗，包括中药、针灸及外敷中药等，疼痛明显减轻，自己高兴地说道，终于可以安稳地睡觉了。

但是没过多久，张女士出现狂躁、疼痛、坐立不安，甚至出现想要从高楼跳下去之类的家人不能理解的举动。原来这是吗啡类药物成瘾后的表现。给她服用吗啡后，症状缓解，但不久就再度复发，又要再服吗啡类西药，这样用药量越来越大，不良反应也越来越强。

也有一些患者，疼痛程度并不严重，但是即使无痛，也每日定时服用止痛药，这样的结果是造成了耐药性、成瘾性越来越大，不良反应也越来越多。我们认为，这样的情况用中医药治疗更为理想。

中医学认为，癌症的疼痛是因为气血阻滞不通所致。中医古籍中有"不通则痛，通则不痛"的观点。气滞血瘀、毒邪蕴积、痰湿凝滞等都会造成不通。因此，治疗癌症疼痛要根据病情而选用活血化瘀、疏肝理气、散结解毒、补阳益阴等治疗方法。

疼痛是癌症的严重病征，要想根本治愈，还是要治本，即治疗肿瘤。中医药有些方剂只是为疼痛不是非常剧烈、没有对西药止痛药成瘾、预约等候需时且精神及生活都尚正常的患者应急而用。癌症疼痛的原因很复杂，有时并不是一个药方就可以解决的。

从中医药对癌症疼痛的治疗来说，本人认为：

（1）不要轻视天然疗法，不要认为只有吗啡等强烈西药才能治癌痛。本书中所附的病案中，治好癌痛的例子很多。应该重视中医药治疗癌症疼痛的研究。

（2）晚期癌症患者使用强力止痛西药的宗旨是减少疼痛，以舒缓痛苦。随着对癌症患者的有效治疗，使患者生活质量和生存时间得以提高、延长，就不得不考虑耐药性、成瘾性等严重不良反应和由其产生的恶劣影响了。

患者消瘦要调理

癌症患者常见消瘦的主要原因是消耗太过。癌细胞与正常组织细胞争夺必需的生存物质。癌细胞快速地生长、增殖、扩散，其掠夺性和疯狂性严重破坏了人体的正常新陈代谢，癌细胞摄取生命必需物质的速度和量，是正常细胞无法比拟的，因此使得患者日益消瘦和虚弱。

癌组织能够产生和释放毒素，可导致患者不思饮食、发热，呈现慢性消耗的状态。有些肿瘤容易引起慢性出血，如消化系统肿瘤、食管癌、胃癌、肠癌等。慢性出血、进食困难、消化吸收障碍等，就会使患者日趋消瘦。肿瘤治疗过程中，例如化疗、放疗，造成骨髓抑制、造血功能障碍等，也是消瘦的主要原因之一。

有的医生要求患者什么都吃，尽量增加营养，其实是需要进一步斟酌的，下面来分析这个问题。

首先，世上各种各样可以吃的东西，本身都有着其自然的属性和特点。用中医理论来讲，首先要考虑到食物的功能特点、性味和归经。例如羊肉是热性食物，热性体质者最好不吃。有发热、牙痛、小便短黄等上火症状者，食后会加重病情。绿豆、苦瓜是寒性食物。如果某人四肢冰冷，腹泻畏寒，吃了这样的食物也会生病或加重病情。

人本身的体质有寒、热、阴、阳等不同的属性，应该用合适的食物和药物来配合调理，才能够健康长寿，而不是用不适合的食物和药物来对抗。好像火上加油，雪上加霜，常人都受不住，更何况是癌症患者呢！所以，什么都可以吃的说法是不对的。

有关大量增加营养的问题。营养过剩导致癌症高发，长期热量过剩以及脂肪、动物蛋白的摄取过多会造成人体代谢紊乱，晚期消瘦的癌症患者，不适合也没有能力消化和吸收此类食物，尤忌每日大鱼大肉，以避免肿瘤细胞摄取过多营养而迅速生长。

"发物"也是要注意避免的。发物指不适当的，能加重病情的食物。民间流传有徐达之死的传说。相传明朝开国大将徐达背部生了一个大疮，郎中看过后嘱咐切忌鸭、鹅类发物。而皇帝却赐给他烧鹅全宴以示慰问，结果徐达食后毒发而死。不管典故真假，不适当的食物会加重病情却是真的。癌症患者适合吃比较清淡、容易消化和吸收的食物，以调养胃气，扶正祛邪。

综上所述，癌症患者的饮食，既不能大量增加动物蛋白、避免发物，又要吃得好以便增强体质、战胜病魔。建议饮食清淡、多样化，以容易消化和吸收的五谷、蔬菜、水果、豆类等为主，还应重视辨证择食，吃适合自己、有益于自己的食物。

夫妻癌现象

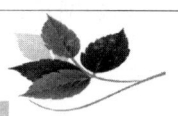

"夫妻癌"即是夫妻两人同时患癌，这种现象越来越普遍。夫妻癌与遗传因素无关，这进一步说明生活习惯、环境及社会因素是患癌的一个非常重要的因素。

长期一起生活的夫妻，兴趣、爱好、生活习惯、起居及心理因素相近，而且互相影响。夫妻两人同住一屋、同睡一床、长期一起作息、一起进食，生活方式相近。例如一起抽烟或一个人抽烟，另一人就被动吸烟；吃得过咸过甜，过于辛辣、刺激；长期食陈旧、腌制食物；长期饮酒；长期不合理的饮食结构；不合理的烹饪方法；长期紧张或焦虑等，都可能逐渐影响双方的健康。

一些细菌病毒的感染，也在共同生活中互相传播。例如某些病毒感染与胃癌、肝癌等有关联。若夫妻其中一方得了癌症，另一方精神上也会出现压力，导致免疫功能下降，或长期生活在紧张焦虑的环境中，或者一方不良的因素，损害对方。以及还有许多未被发现、认识尚不足的因素，都推动着夫妻癌现象节节攀升。

夫妻癌的增长数字，颇值得重视。根据上海世界卫生组织、上海癌症研究合作中心统计，每一百对死亡的夫妻中，大约有五对是"夫妻癌"。

注意改正不良的生活习惯，注意发现和纠正周围环境和与生活密切相关的各种不良因素，有助于减少夫妻癌的发生。

审证求因治疗癌性胸腹水

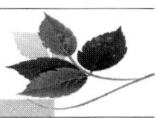

癌性胸腹水和水肿是由多方面的原因所造成。例如，乳腺癌患者术后的上肢水肿，是由于手术的切割和大面积淋巴廓清的程序，使得腋窝淋巴引流通路阻断，大量含蛋白质的淋巴液滞留在组织间隙，血管内外及肢体渗透压梯度减少，导致大量液体进入组织间隙造成上肢水肿。

肿瘤压迫也是很多患者出现水肿的常见原因。血液循环和淋巴液回流因肿瘤的压迫被阻塞。此外，肝癌等恶性肿瘤出现下肢水肿的主要原因还有腹部肿瘤或腹水、癌栓阻塞，其压迫下肢静脉，使静脉回流受阻。

癌症的营养不良，一般认为白蛋白过低也会水肿。中医学认为，各种原因导致的体内水液运行障碍，都可引起局部或全身的水肿。

胸腹水是中晚期癌症患者常见的并发症，会严重影响患者的生活质量和生存期。有些甚至出现心包积液等，这些都有可能危及生命。而频繁的外科治疗手段，例如放水、抽水等，仅能使患者暂时轻松一些，但容易导致胸腹水更快、量更多地滋生，全身也更快衰竭，临床这样的案例很多，可见这些手段及某些药物的不当使用，会造成类似的恶性循环，使患者出现乏力、周身酸痛、恶心及积水不消的情况。治疗无效的原因通常有以下几种。

（1）重复抽放胸腹水，可导致胸腹水产生速度更快，一般三天之后，积水就会再次出现，约七天便会增至之前的水平。

（2）患者体内因抽胸腹水造成的蛋白流失，可能导致低蛋白血症，使患者病情变得更差，身体消瘦虚弱。

（3）抽胸腹水容易增加感染机会。

（4）抽胸腹水可能导致胸膜、胸腔等部位逐渐粘连形成包裹性积液，会使患者出现咳嗽、气促、胸痛、呼吸困难等症状，从而使治疗更加困难。

（5）腔内注射药物易使患者出现呕吐、胸痛、腹痛、发热、寒热、白细胞下降等情况。重复腔内注射，还可能导致呼吸困难，引起腹痛、肠坏死等。

综上所述，这样的治疗方式弊多于利，更可能导致病情转差，生活质量下降，甚至失去了与癌对抗的能力。

中医治疗胸腹水和水肿有补肾助阳、健脾利湿、峻下逐水等多种方法，临床运用得当，注重治本，则会有良好的效果。

抗癌治疗与带瘤生存

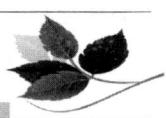

人人都想有健康的身体，但常常事与愿违，不同年龄的人都可能患上各式各样的疾病，如心脏病、高血压、糖尿病、肺炎、胃病等。虽然随着医学研究不断进步，许多疾病受到一定程度的控制，但是直至目前，癌症仍是发病率越来越高且死亡率极高的疾病。当前对癌症的治疗方法主要有化疗、放射治疗（放疗）、手术。但是在相当多的情况下，这些治疗的效果并不理想，许多患者抱着生存的希望，极力忍受这些治疗带来的极大痛苦，到头来还是失去了生命。有些患者在治疗过程中就离世，有些即使坚持完成了这些治疗，但不久就因为复发、转移或机体过度衰竭而离世……这样的例子太多了，以至于人们都以为癌症就是绝症。

癌症不是绝症

其实，癌症不是绝症，患癌也不等于死亡，关键是要在治疗方法上去改变、去革新。传统医学在治疗疾病时，会先对患者的整体状况进行详细的辨别。例如，有的患者身体过分虚弱，便不推荐其接受化疗、放疗，患者过分虚弱的病体，已承受不起任何打击，否则只能雪上加霜、加速死亡。中医药的治疗原则，完全不同于化疗和放疗。抗癌中医药治疗首先使患者的病情稳定下来，使肿瘤生长、发展的速度缓和下来；其次，使患者过度虚损的身体，逐渐恢复过来；再次，使发展迅猛、威胁生命的癌症恶魔，转变成为可以控制的、状态稳定的、对生命没有严重威胁的慢性病，以为进一步抗癌治疗赢得宝贵时间。

实际上，我们已经在许多抗癌中医药治疗案例中做到了这一点。许多患者来就诊时已经气息奄奄，医院已明确告知家人无法医治了。但经过完全不同的方法治疗后，患者病情逐步得以控制和好转。虽然肿瘤并未很快消失，但抗癌中医药治疗为患者赢得了带病生存的机会和进一步治疗的时间，很多患者由此走向康复。

这种全新的中医药治疗方法，需要进一步研究，才能更加完善，才能救助更多的癌症患者，也期望社会各界伸出援手，支持中医药抗癌研究的进一步发展。

癌症复发和转移勿放弃

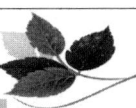

癌症的重要特点就是容易复发和转移，这也是恶性肿瘤与良性肿瘤的重要区别。绝大多数的癌症晚期患者有癌症复发和转移。尽管做了手术、放疗、化疗，但癌症的复发和转移的概率并没有因此而降低。

常见到有些癌症患者术后（或未进行手术）不停地进行化疗，稍有停顿，癌指数就会上升。还有一些患者即使一直做化疗和靶向治疗，癌指数也继续增高，肿瘤继续增大，甚至出现新的肿瘤、新的转移灶等。长期这样下去往往使患者身体极度衰弱，免疫功能低下，相当多的人难以承受。

在这些情况下，中医药治疗是一个很好的选择。较早期的患者，如果及早用中医药治疗，往往能很好地控制肿瘤生长，降低肿瘤复发和转移的概率。晚期的患者用中医药治疗，同样也能起到一定的疗效。

举个例子：李先生，于2009年2月出现腹胀、胃口差，接着出现了黄疸、水肿，医院检查结果证明确实患了肝癌。在惊慌之下，他们天天找不同的医生、专家，去不同的医院、诊所就诊，然而所有的回答都一样，就是太晚期了，肿瘤很大，腹腔、骨、肺等部位都有转移，无法做手术，即使是化疗也仅有 0.5% 的希望，明确说来，他的生命只余几星期了。

在这种走投无路的情况下，李先生只有选择抗癌中医药治疗了。他认真服用中药，至今已近三年，期间也发生过几次严重的问题，并有腹痛、腰痛、胃口差、发热等症状，但经及时的抗癌中医药治疗，都有惊无险地度过去了。现在他每天能在服用中药的同时正常地工作和生活。他和家人对继续治疗都很有信心。大量事实表明，中医药治疗各种癌症是有效的，它的优势表现在以下几个方面：

（1）预防肿瘤复发和转移。早期患者及时治疗，效果更明显。

（2）控制肿瘤复发和转移。如果出现肿瘤的复发和转移，中医药治疗可使病灶逐渐平息、稳定，控制肿瘤的生长速度，缓解相关的严重症状。晚期患者，只要治疗正确，也能够正常生活。

（3）使病情长期稳定，转移病灶，使肿瘤逐渐缩小以至消失。

（4）进一步的研究正在进行中，深入研究其实质，有利于取得更好的治疗效果，并进一步揭示复发、转移的机制。

中医药治癌新观念

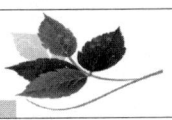

中医药治癌和西医治癌有很多不同之处,中医药治癌有以下几个特点。

以人为本

中医药治疗的核心是以人为本,注重患者的全身状态。如果患者的身体非常虚弱,就需要优先调治。而西医更重视肿瘤本身,治疗以抗肿瘤为主。

注重整体

中医重视整体的调治,认为肿瘤只是整体失常的局部表现,而西医更重视对肿瘤的局部治疗。但是如果不重整体,"杀敌一千,自损一万",将身体治垮了,就失去了治疗的意义。

无毒无害

中医药治疗不是攻击性的治疗。西医的化疗、放疗、手术都是攻击性，以杀死癌细胞为目的的治疗。患者常越来越虚弱，甚至会出现脏器功能衰竭等情况。而中医是以养生、扶助正气为主，更重视培养人体本身的抗病能力，发挥人体本身的抗癌消瘤功能，使患者通过逐渐增强体质来发挥最大优势抗癌。然而有些中医药治癌的方式笔者并不赞同，比如使用许多有毒的药物来以毒攻毒。化疗、放疗已经够毒了，如果化疗后肿瘤还没被控制，再用毒药来以毒攻毒，一是无济于事，二是患者难以承受，所以扶正祛邪、养生抗癌才是恰当的中医药治癌方法。

辨证施治

中医主张根据患者实际情况决定治疗方案，即因人而异辨证施治。而不是不停地一个化疗紧接一个化疗，又再接一个放疗，再加上靶向药物这样的治疗方式，使患者没有喘息和体能恢复机会的治疗。

养生为要

癌症得到控制并不是万事大吉，之后仍存在许多潜在的危险。稍有不慎，便可能发生肿瘤的复发或转移。想使病情稳定，就需要较长时间全面调理，注重养生，随时关注已出现或可能出现的问题，及时调理，平衡气血阴阳，达到长治久安。

不言放弃

许多晚期患者生命垂危，有的经大医院、高级医生判定死刑，有的经判定只剩下几个月、几周、甚至几天的生命，他们经过抗癌中医药的合理治疗，都重拾了信心，生活了更长时间。所以不要轻言放弃，用乐观、耐心、勇气、信念和坚持治疗来征服癌症。

带病延年养生长寿

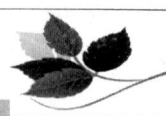

在广西巴马的长寿村，我们对能够见到的每一位百岁老人都进行了详细的了解和调查，并从现代医学和中医学两个角度，为他们做了身体检查。

除了赞叹他们的生命长青外，我们尤其注意到他们在一生中共有的生活经历及特点，主要有以下方面：①粗茶淡饭；②素食为主；③新鲜原始食物为主；④生活艰苦；⑤空气清新；⑥生活环境比较原始；⑦很少看病吃西药；⑧终生劳动不息；⑨有较强的抗压能力；⑩每人都有病，带病延年。

这些百岁老人，经历了漫长的岁月风霜，大多都患有胃病、腰腿痛等，他们中的几乎每位都可见到关节变形，有的腰已不能伸直，只能弯腰九十度行走。所见的媒体报道，都没有提过这些百岁老人的病情，而我们作为医生，在为他们做体检的同时，也为他们开方治病，因为他们全部有病痛，在一位106岁的老人的颈部还发现了肿瘤。

这不得不使人感慨，这些百岁老人如果生活在富裕的城市，也许早就被送进了医院，使用了大量的抗生素、激素，并长期服用了很多化学药物，破坏了自己的抗病能力。同时每日的山珍海味、大鱼大肉，会使身体发福、血管硬化、循环阻滞，毒素充斥全身；空调的温度，会使他们丧失了与恶劣环境抗争的能力；舒适的生活，会使他们失去承受精神打击和高度压力的能力；人们之间的竞争、尔虞我诈，会使他们失眠紧张，以及产生不满、嫉妒、憎恨、愤怒的不良情绪。对于金钱的无休止的欲望，会使他们失去快乐轻松的心情。对于现代化物质的享受，会使他们抛弃晨露阳光、和风细雨的自然之神的馈赠。

其实，他们不是不想吃肉，而是没得吃；他们不是不想休息享清福，而是不劳动就不能生存。这些恶劣的环境、贫困的生活、清新的空气、宽容处世的态度，正是天地给予生命的最丰厚的礼物，使得他们长命百岁。

值得注意的是，有些百岁老人的子孙，进了城，有了工作，生活比他们不知好多少倍，但却早于他们而离世，说明遗传因素并不是最重要的、决定性的因素。这些百岁老人的经历，使我们信心大增，他们在那样贫困恶劣的环境中，仍可以带病长寿，在当今，更多的人享有优良的医疗保证，带病延年、养生长寿应该不是梦想。

下篇

抗癌治验录

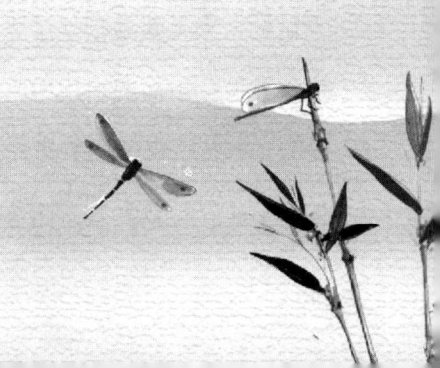

病案 1
抗癌明星，百岁寿星

杨太太是我们的老患者，也是名副其实的大明星——抗癌明星和百岁寿星。杨太太今年已经104岁了，这天，她精神饱满、腰板挺直地走进诊所，一进门就与在候诊的患者们打招呼，还拿出自己亲手制作的馒头，与大家分享。香港人以米饭为主食，馒头是稀罕物，又见是百岁寿星制作的，大家都争先恐后去抢，围坐在老寿星身旁，想多沾得一些老寿星的正气、喜气。但是一些新来的患者还不知道，杨太太是我们的抗癌明星。

20多年前，就是1994年，杨太太被查出患了乳腺癌，已有淋巴转移，当时医院要求进行放疗和化疗，但是杨太太身体很差，每日精神萎靡、弱不禁风、进食很少、消瘦、头晕、胸部肿胀。她想，如果行化疗和放疗，这条老命一定会搭进去，于是杨太太果断地拒绝了医生、儿孙、家人的劝告，坚决不做化疗和放疗，而要求用中医药的生命修复法治疗。之后她听从医嘱，坚持认真服用中药，学习养生，就这样20多年过去了，如今104岁的她比20多年前更健康、更有精神。治病的过程其实并不一帆风顺,在2~3年前,她的乳腺癌在腋下、乳下等部位复发,胸部多处可摸到肿块,症见胸胁逆满,呃气多,心情郁闷,舌淡红,脉弦细,她除了认真吃药外,还主动要求给增加针灸等治疗方法。有时病人多,她也不着急,让别人先看,说自己年老了,反正没什么事,多等会也没关系。就这样到现在经检查,复发的肿瘤全部消失,她快乐健康地享受天伦之乐。

治则:固本补肾,舒肝散结。

常用中药:熟地黄、鹿茸片、瓜蒌、王不留行、皂角刺、八月札、山慈菇、土鳖虫、枸杞子、淫羊藿等,散结粉,同中药汤剂一起冲服。

患者年老体衰，扶正固本补肾势在必需。熟地黄、枸杞子、淫羊藿等为补肾扶正而设，鹿茸片补阳益精，又是阴疽常用。皂角刺、山慈菇、瓜蒌等为治疗乳腺肿瘤常用，土鳖虫逐瘀通乳。诸药同用，共奏固本补肾、疏肝散结之功。

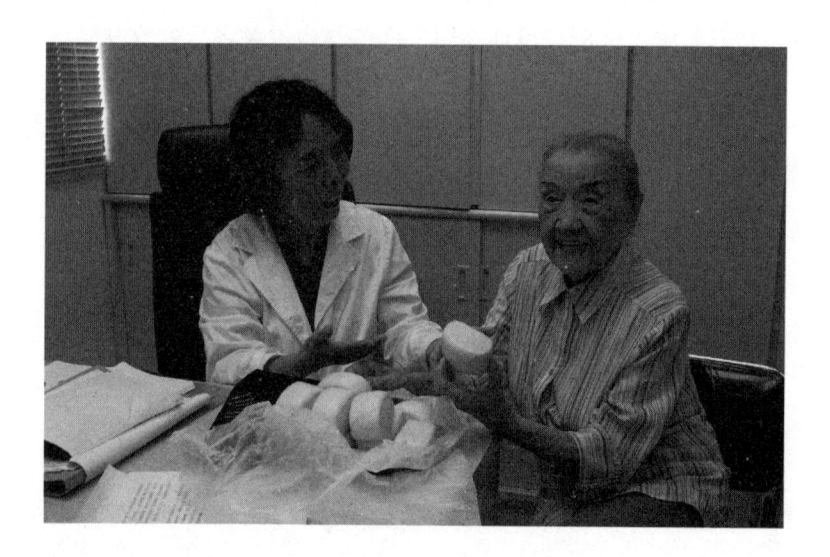

病案 2
晚期鼻咽癌康复

2006年，冯先生三十七岁，正值青春年华，家庭事业都一帆风顺。有一天，他使用电脑很晚未睡，突然感到前额有些胀痛，一低头，见有鲜血滴在地上，他很震惊，急忙照镜子，原来在流鼻血。

冯先生想，一定是熬夜上了火，喝点凉茶就会没事了。但是在其后的一个月，冯先生尽管喝了不少凉茶，他的鼻子仍经常流血，有时量还很多，难以止住，同时伴有鼻塞、头痛等不适症状出现，他只好到医院看医生。经检查发现，他的鼻腔内有个较大的肿瘤，医生要求取活组织检查并作正电子扫描。

数周后，检查报告证实冯先生患了鼻咽癌，肿瘤为未分化型，恶性程度很高，且已是晚期。CT检查报告指出，他的鼻咽癌已生长至后鼻孔、筛骨、蝶骨、左眼眶、鼻咽顶部、颈部及颈椎等部位，最危险的是肿瘤距离视神经仅有五毫米，也就是说，冯先生的鼻咽癌向颅骨及颈部等有较广泛转移，同时还有失明的危险。西医安排冯先生做放疗，并表明病情已属晚期，即使做了放疗，复发、转移和失明的可能性都很大。

冯先生决定用各种方法与癌病抗争，在接受西医放疗的同时，进行生命修复抗癌中医药治疗，希望能够找到对抗晚期恶性肿瘤的办法。

治则：疏肝解郁，养阴解毒，散结抗癌。

常用中药：柴胡、黄芩、鱼腥草、夏枯草、重楼、麦冬、露蜂房、山慈菇、玄参、石斛、牡蛎等，另配制消瘤粉与汤药同服。

患者属邪毒炽盛，阴精耗损，虚实并具。放射线是热毒，造成对患者正气的损伤和阴津耗损，如单纯攻邪，会致阴精、正气更虚，故采用补虚攻邪之法。柴胡、黄芩清少阳之经，鱼腥草、夏枯草清热解毒、疏郁，麦冬、石斛养阴生津、露蜂房、山慈菇、重楼，散结解毒抗癌。重楼苦，微寒，清热解毒，用于热毒炽盛。露蜂房攻毒疗疮，与重楼配合使用，二者相辅相成，有明显解毒抗癌功效。玄参与石斛、牡蛎配合，滋阴解毒、软坚散结。对于头颅的瘰疬淋巴结转移肿瘤常多用而效佳。

冯先生每日坚持服用中药，每周都按时就诊，风雨不改。至2007年5月，冯先生的努力有了成效。检查报告指出肿瘤已全部消失，此后他继续服用中药，生活恢复正常。

用药两年没复发转移

两年后，即 2009 年 7 月冯先生再去检查，结果也没有发生令人忧虑的复发和转移。时至今日，距冯先生被确诊为鼻咽癌并多发颅部、颈部等转移已过十一年时间，肿瘤也没有复发和转移，他的生活和工作都保持正常。他于 2006 年至 2009 年坚持每日用抗癌中医药治疗，其后间断服用中药，再后来只是偶然到来，用中医药调理身体。

鼻咽癌是一种常见的恶性肿瘤，发生扩散和转移后，可预期往后情况会很差。冯先生的鼻咽癌已发生严重的扩散和骨、淋巴等转移，经治疗后现已正常生活十一年。这进一步说明肿瘤扩散转移后，患者和家人、医生都不应轻言放弃。

诊疗记录

2006 年 9 月 1 日 CT 检查报告证实鼻咽癌，并有较广泛的颅骨及周围骨转移，已接近侵犯视神经。

附：患者检查报告

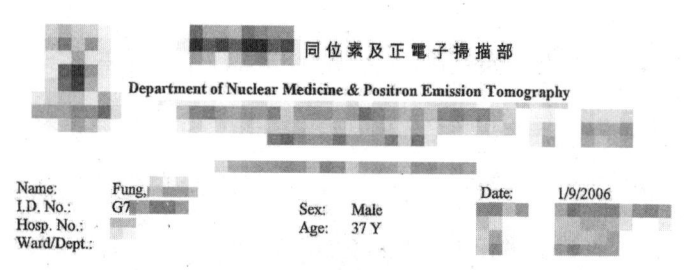

同位素及正電子掃描部
Department of Nuclear Medicine & Positron Emission Tomography

Name:	Fung,	Date:	1/9/2006
I.D. No.:	G7	Sex:	Male
Hosp. No.:		Age:	37 Y
Ward/Dept.:			

POSITRON EMISSION TOMOGRAPHY
(^{18}F-FDG ONCOLOGY)

History:

A 37 year-old gentleman presented with left epistaxis. Biopsy on 23/8/2006 confirmed nasopharyngeal carcinoma. Clinical and MRI showed disease in left nasal cavity extending up to the inferior aspect of ethmoidal-sphenoid junction medial to left bony orbit, left NP sidewall, roof of nasopharynx and neck is clear. PET scan is now performed for staging. Body weight, appetite and sleep are normal. Bowel movement and urination normal. No bone pain, no cough, no night sweat. Non-smoker, non-drinker. No history of hepatitis or tuberculosis. Did not take any herbs. Took boiled lingzhi for a few years for ~10 times a few years ago. No family history of TB and cancer.

Procedures:

Fasting blood glucose at 10:40 was 5.7 mmol/l. 60 mg Spasmonal was given p.o. 15 min before ^{18}FDG. 12.8 mCi of ^{18}F-FDG was injected at 10:50. PET-CT scan from base of skull to groin was performed at 11:52 (62 minutes after injection).

Findings:

SUVmax = Standardized Uptake Value Maximum
SUVavg = Standardized Uptake Value Average

Liver tissue normal reference uptake has a SUVmax of 2.86 and a SUVavg of 2.33. Delayed PET-CT SUVmax 2.11 and SUVavg 2.01.

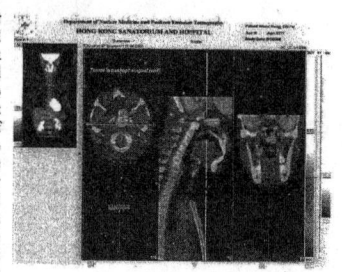

A hypermetabolic mass can be seen in the anterior nasopharyngeal roof. This is consistent with clinical diagnosis of nasopharyngeal carcinoma(3.6 cm W x 3.1 cm H x 4.9 cm D, SUVmax 11.76, delayed SUVmax 12.99). The tumor anteriorly extends into the left posterior nasal choana and cephalically it protrudes cephalically into the inferior part of ethmoid sinus. Laterally it is situated proximal to the left supra-orbital fissure. There is no definite bony erosion can be identified. Inferiorly the tumor is at the level of upper border of C1 ring, and anteriorly in the nasal choana is just cephalic to the left nasal inferior concha. No definite hypermetabolic lymph node can be seen. There is some mild asymmetric with a mild increase on the left side of the left jugulo-digastric node just posterior medial to the angle of left mandible. There is some tiny lymph node seen there more than the contralateral side.

Both lungs appear clear and the mediastinum shows normal physiological activities. The cardiac muscle shows normal increased uptake. The liver shows uniform uptake without any focal area of

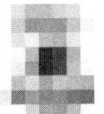

Department of Nuclear Medicine & Positron Emission Tomography

hypermetabolism. The adrenal glands appear normal. There is no abnormal abdominal para-aortic lymph node. The bowel shows some physiological activity in the muscle of the intestine. There is no abnormal pelvic uptake. Both groins appear normal with no abnormal lymphadenopathy. There is no abnormal uptake in the prostate area.

Impression:

1. The findings are consistent with the clinical diagnosis of nasopharyngeal carcinoma situating in the nasopharyngeal roof area. The tumor anteriorly extends into the left posterior nasal choana and also cephalic protruding into the left ethmoid sinus. Laterally, the tumor is in close proximity to the optic nerve in the superior orbital fissure. There is no definite osseous erosion. The inferior border of the tumor would be about the plane of C1.
2. No macroscopic metastatic lymph node can be seen but some tiny lymph nodes in the left jugulo-digastric node show mild asymmetrical activity increased on the left side. Thus microscopic metastasis to the left jugulo-digastric nodes posterior medial to the angle of mandible cannot be completely excluded.
3. No distant metastasis can be seen.

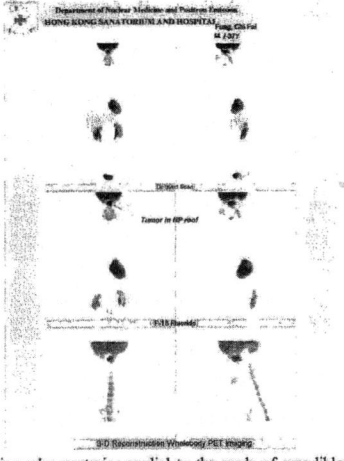

MBBS(HK), DABNuM, DABPed
Consultant in Nuclear Medicine

同位素及正電子掃描部
Department of Nuclear Medicine & Positron Emission Tomography

Name: Fung, 馮
I.D. No.: G7
Hosp. No.: O.1
Ward/Dept.:

Sex: Male
Age: 39 Y

Date: 24/1/2008

POSITRON EMISSION TOMOGRAPHY
(^{18}F-FDG ONCOLOGY)

History:

A 39 year-old gentleman with nasopharyngeal carcinoma diagnosed in 8/2006, status post chemoradiation therapy, last radiation therapy completed in 11/2006, for follow-up evaluation. Prior PET scan of 31/5/2007 was negative.

Patient is currently asymptomatic.

Radiopharmaceutical: 12.2 mCi F-18 Fluorodeoxyglucose (^{18}FDG) injected intravenously.

Findings:

Limited whole body CT transmission and PET emission imaging began at 100 minutes after radiopharmaceutical administration (blood glucose 5.8 mmol/l), spanning a region from base of skull to upper thigh. 60 mg Spasmonal was given p.o. 15 min before ^{18}FDG administration.

Liver tissue normal reference uptake has a SUVmax of 2.12

There are no abnormal focal ^{18}FDG activities in the nasopharynx. There are no ^{18}FDG-avid enlarged lymph nodes in the head and neck region. There is mild asymmetric ^{18}FDG activity in the right vocal cord, a non-specific finding.

There are no hypermetabolic enlarged lymph nodes in the mediastinum or the axillae. Bilateral lung fields are clear with no evidence of pulmonary nodules.

In the abdomen, there is normal diffuse low-grade ^{18}FDG activity in the liver and spleen. There are no abnormal focal ^{18}FDG activities in the pancreas and the GI tract. No hypermetabolic lymph nodes are seen in the celiac axis or the retroperitoneal space of the abdomen and pelvis.

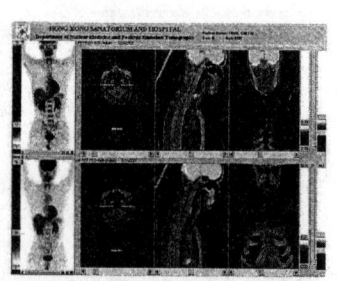

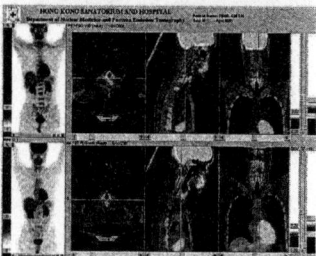

The rest of the visualized structures show normal radiotracer activity. There is no abnormal focal uptake in the bony structures to suggest osseous metastasis.

抗癌治验录 下篇

Department of Nuclear Medicine & Positron Emission Tomography

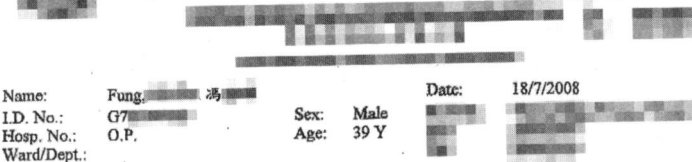

同位素及正電子掃描部

Name:	Fung, ███ 冯 ███	Date:	18/7/2008
I.D. No.:	G7███	Sex:	Male
Hosp. No.:	O.P.	Age:	39 Y
Ward/Dept.:			

POSITRON EMISSION TOMOGRAPHY
(^{18}F-FDG ONCOLOGY)

History:

A 39 year-old gentleman with nasopharyngeal carcinoma diagnosed in 2006, status post chemoradiation therapy completed in 11/2006 for follow-up evaluation. He has been clinically asymptomatic.

Radiopharmaceutical: 11.3 mCi F-18 Fluorodeoxyglucose (^{18}FDG) injected intravenously.

Findings:

Limited whole body CT transmission and PET emission imaging began at 76 minutes after radiopharmaceutical administration (blood glucose 5.4 mmol/l), spanning a region from base of skull to upper thigh. 60 mg Spasmonal was given p.o. 15 min before ^{18}FDG administration.

Liver tissue normal reference uptake has a SUVmax of 2.95.

Comparison is made with prior PET scan dated 24/1/2008.

There is mild decreased ^{18}FDG activity in the left side of the nasopharynx, unchanged since the prior study and consistent with post-treatment changes. There are no ^{18}FDG-avid or enlarged lymph nodes in bilateral neck and axillae.

Bilateral lung fields are clear with no pulmonary nodules. There are no hypermetabolic or enlarged lymph nodes in the mediastinum.

There is normal diffuse ^{18}FDG activity in the liver and spleen. There are no hypermetabolic or enlarged lymph nodes in the celiac axis, retroperitoneal space of the abdomen and pelvis, and bilateral inguinal regions. There are no abnormal focal uptake in the pancreas and the GI tract. The adrenals are normal in size and non-^{18}FDG-avid.

The rest of the visualized structures show normal radiotracer activity. There are no abnormal focal uptake in the bony structures to suggest osseous metastasis.

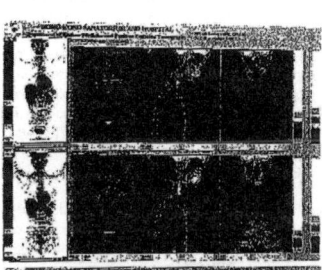

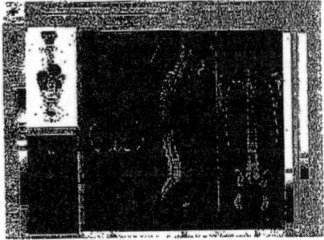

同位素及正電子掃描部
Department of Nuclear Medicine & Positron Emission Tomography

DOCTOR'S COPY

Name:	Fung, 馮	Sex:	Male	Date:	29/07/2009
I.D. No.:	G7	Age:	40 Y		
Hosp. No.:	O.P.				
Ward/Dept.:					

POSITRON EMISSION TOMOGRAPHY
(^{18}F-FDG ONCOLOGY)

History:

40 year-old gentleman with nasopharyngeal carcinoma diagnosed in 2006, status post chemoradiation therapy completed in 11/2006, for follow-up evaluation. He has been clinically asymptomatic.

Radiopharmaceutical: 12.4 mCi F-18 Fluorodeoxyglucose (^{18}FDG) injected intravenously.

Findings:

Limited whole body CT transmission and PET emission imaging began at 59 minutes after radiopharmaceutical administration (blood glucose 5.5 mmol/l), spanning a region from base of skull to upper thigh. 60 mg Spasmonal was given p.o. 15 min before ^{18}FDG administration.

Liver tissue normal reference uptake has a SUVmax of 2.36.

Comparison is made with prior PET scan dated 18/07/2008.

There is no abnormal focal ^{18}FDG activity in the nasopharynx. There are no ^{18}FDG-avid or enlarged lymph nodes in bilateral neck and axillae. There is mild asymmetric increased ^{18}FDG activity in the left base of tongue that is within normal physiologic variation. This was also seen in PET scans of 01/2008 and 07/2008 and has been stable.

Bilateral lung fields are clear with no pulmonary nodules. There are no hypermetabolic or enlarged lymph nodes in the mediastinum and bilateral hilar regions.

In the abdomen, there is normal diffuse ^{18}FDG activity in the liver and spleen. There are no hypermetabolic lymph nodes in the celiac axis, retroperitoneal space of the abdomen and pelvis. There are no abnormal focal ^{18}FDG activities in the pancreas, kidneys and the GI tract. Adrenals are normal.

The rest of the visualized structures show normal radiotracer activity. There are no hypermetabolic bone lesions to suggest osseous metastasis.

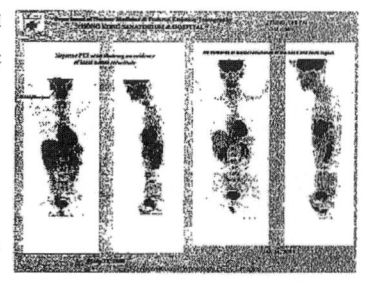

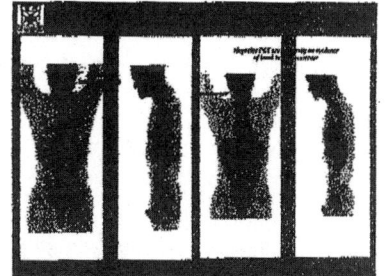

抗癌治验录 下篇

同位素及正電子掃描部
Department of Nuclear Medicine & Positron Emission Tomography

Impression:

1. Negative PET scan showing no evidence of local tumor recurrence.
2. There is no evidence of lymph node or distant metastasis.

Thank you very much, ███, for your referral.

M.B,B.S.(H.K.),A.B.I.M.,A.B.N.M.,F.R.C.R.(U.K.),F.H.K.C.R.,F.H.K.A.M.(Radiology)
Department of Nuclear Medicine & P.E.T.

同位素及正電子掃描部
Department of Nuclear Medicine & Positron Emission Tomography

Impression:

1. Negative PET scan showing no evidence of local tumor recurrence.
2. There is no evidence of lymph node or distant metastasis.

Thank you very much, ███, for your referral.

M.B,B.S.(H.K.),A.B.I.M.,A.B.N.M.,F.R.C.R.(U.K.),F.H.K.C.R.,
F.H.K.A.M.(Radiology)
Department of Nuclear Medicine & P.E.T.

病案 3
降服肺癌脑转移

2007年8月，陈先生经检查发现患了肺癌，且为第三期肺癌，他按照医生的安排，翌月开始化疗，一直化疗到年底，但疗效不好，于是换化疗药物，再继续化疗。

2008年2月，陈先生的病情加重，出现了胸腔积液、肿瘤纵隔及胸膜转移，至2009年6月检查发现肺癌脑转移。

医院的医生跟他解释，肺癌脑转移是最末期的严重情况，除再行放疗外，无法可医，而放疗效果也不理想。在这种无法可医的情况下陈先生于2009年7月初寻求生命修复抗癌中医药治疗续命。当时陈先生症见头晕、头痛、胸闷、气喘、多痰、咳嗽、纳差、无力，精神状态很差，面色苍白，舌淡红，脉沉细。

治疗原则：补益脾肾，攻逐痰结。

常用中药：党参、茯苓、泽泻、鱼脑石、青礞石、山慈菇、黄药子、淫羊藿、菟丝子、制甘遂、大戟、葶苈子，散结丸、消瘤粉同时服用。

患者体内水液代谢失调有脑水肿、胸腔积液，又有肺的肿瘤和脑的转移瘤，辨证得痰浊结聚。虽肿瘤上移至脑，但原发灶在肺，加紧对原发癌灶的治疗，就是对脑转移的有效治疗。

党参、茯苓、泽泻补气健脾，化痰行水。淫羊藿、菟丝子，除了补肾，强健水运之外共同健运中焦，温补下焦。鱼脑石、青礞石、山慈菇、黄药子，涤痰，软坚散结，抗癌。制甘遂、大戟、葶苈子为攻逐水饮而设。

抽水次数日渐减少

至2010年5月，陈先生经CT检查，脑转移病灶已消失，但仍需继续治疗肺部肿瘤、胸腔积液等。他因胸膜纵隔转移，以前要定期到医院抽水，后来逐渐减少抽水次数，最后更是不再需要抽水了。

陈先生的病情逐渐稳定，生活也恢复正常。算起来，他自检查发现脑转移，至2016年随访时止，已有七年；发生胸膜纵隔等转移，已有七年；而距发现三期肺癌，已有九年。

一般人都认为，陈先生是不可能生存至今的，特别是发生脑转移后，患者的病情常会迅速恶化，尽管医生和病人、家人想尽各种办法都无济于事。但陈先生经生命修复抗癌中医药治疗后身体、工作得以恢复正常。

服用中药控制病情

抗癌中医药治疗使陈先生的病情逐渐得到控制,并进一步把发展猖狂的癌魔制服。

中医的古典医籍中曾经提到"未可治者,不得其术也"。就是说,如果有什么病不能治疗,是因为没有找到合适的治疗方法;如果找到合适的方法,各种疾病都是可以治疗的。癌症也是一样,我们希望继续深入研究中医药宝库,以便救治更多的生命。

抗癌治验录 **下篇**

诊疗记录

2009年6月22日CT检查证实为肺癌、胸腔积水、肺不张、胸膜转移、纵隔多发淋巴转移，并有脑转移。

2012年11月12日CT检查证实，病情明显好转，肿瘤结节消失，胸腔积水减少，脑转移肿瘤消失。

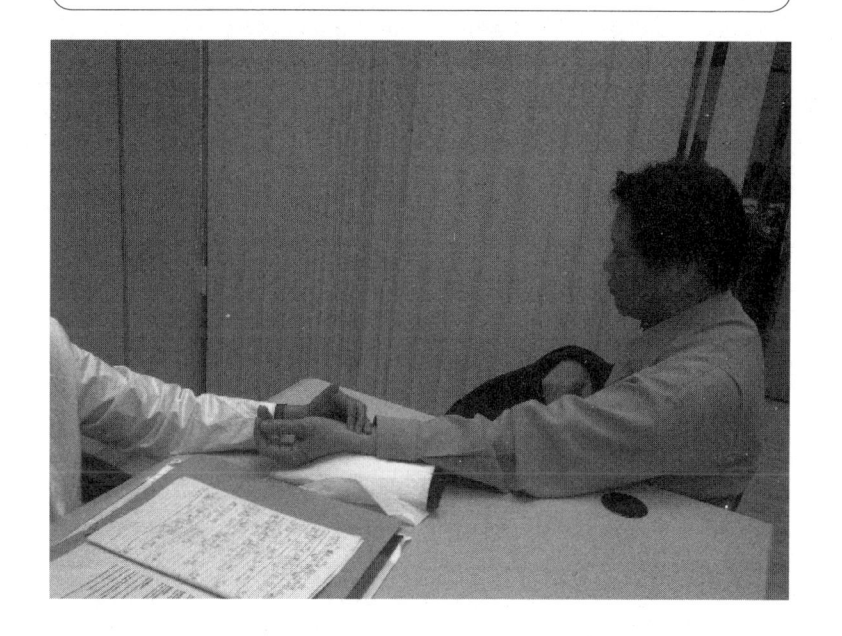

治癌实录 2
中晚期癌症・名家手记

附：患者检查报告

Patient Name	: CHAN		
Sex/Age	: M/ 57	Examination Date :	22/6/2009
		Reported Date :	22/6/2009
Examination	: WHOLE BODY PET CT SCAN		

CT, Brain With IV contrast:
Post contrast scan was performed from skull base to vertex.

There is an enhancing nodule at the left frontal region at 1cm in keeping with metastasis.

There is no other abnormal density or contrast enhancement is detected in the leptomeninges, cerebral or cerebellar hemispheres. No cerebral oedema is seen. There is no deviation of the midline structure.

The ventricles are of normal dimensions. Normal sulcal and gyral pattern is present over both cerebral hemispheres. The pituitary gland and pineal gland are not enlarged. The brainstem and cerebellum are normally defined.

No extra-dural collection or calvarial destruction is observed.

COMMENT: Left frontal solitary metastasis is noted.

Whole Body PET-CT Scan:

Thorax:
There have been previous VATS at the right lung.

There is no evidence of new nodule or abnormal metabolism to suggest local recurrence at the surgical site and right lung.

The calcified granulomata at the right and left lung apices are unchanged. A tiny postinflammatory nodule is found at the anterior segment of RUL which remains unchanged. No new lung nodule is evident. The atelectasis at the RML is unchanged.

The right basal pleural effusion has increased to 6.5cm (image 105), while it was at maximum diameter of 2.7cm. No pleural thickening or FDG uptake is identified. A mildly FDG-avid plaque is noted at the posterobasal region (image 100) of the RLL suspicious of pleural deposit at SUVmax 1.9, with size 1 x 0.7cm.

There is no pericardial effusion observed.

Node (table 1):
There are multiple hypermetabolic nodal deposits developed since last study in the mediastinum. They have SUVmax 3-3.4. Please see table 1 for reference.

No hypermetabolic node is found at the neck, abdomen and pelvis.

Abdomen & Pelvis:
Both adrenals are not enlarged. No abnormal FDG-uptake is present in the adrenals.

Patient Name	: CHAN		
Sex/Age	: M/ 57	Examination Date	: 22/6/2009
		Reported Date	: 22/6/2009
Examination	: WHOLE BODY PET CT SCAN		

No ascites or peritoneal deposit is found.

The liver is not enlarged. The IVC, portal veins and hepatic veins are patent. The biliary tract is not dilated.

There is no hypermetabolic mass detected in spleen, pancreas and kidneys. There is no hydronephrosis or hydroureter present. Normal FDG excretion is noted in both kidneys.

There is no abnormal bowel wall thickening detected. The ileocecal region is of normal calibre.

Urinary bladder is normal. The prostate is enlarged and contains calcification. Ischio-rectal fossae are unremarkable.

Head & Neck Region:
No abnormal soft tissue mass or FDG uptake is evident in the tonsil, thyroid, pharynx, nasopharynx or larynx. The visualised portions of the para-nasal sinuses are clear.

Skeleton:
No hypermetabolic sclerotic or lytic destruction is identified. No abnormal FDG accumulation is observed in the marrow to suggest bone metastasis. There is no pathological fracture or vertebral collapse seen. Minor spinal spondylitic changes are evident.

COMMENT:
Status CA right lung post VATS and chemotherapy.

Nodal recurrence is evident at the mediastinum. No local recurrence is noted at surgical site in the RUL.

The right basal pleural effusion has increased likely to be malignant in nature.

Solitary metastasis is found at the left frontal lobe.

No metastasis is detected at the adrenals, liver, contralateral lung & bones.

Table 1:
New nodal deposits are listed as follow:

Site	Image	Size (cm)	SUV max
Rt peri-oesophageal	83	1.6	3
Subcarinal	89	1.3	3.3
Rt hilar	89	1.3	3.1
Rt hilar	95	1.3	3.4

MBBS (HK), FRCR (UK), FHKCR, FHKAM (Radiology)

治癌实录 2
中晚期癌症・名家手记

Patient Name	: CHAN		
Sex/Age	: M/ 59	Examination Date :	12/11/2010
		Reported Date :	12/11/2010
Examination	: WHOLE BODY PET CT SCAN		

The liver is not enlarged. The IVC, portal veins and hepatic veins are patent. The biliary tract is not dilated.

There is no hypermetabolic mass detected in spleen, pancreas and kidneys. There is no hydronephrosis or hydroureter present. Normal FDG excretion is noted in both kidneys.

There is no abnormal bowel wall thickening detected. The ileocecal region is of normal calibre.

Urinary bladder is normal. The prostate is enlarged and contains calcification. Ischio-rectal fossae are unremarkable.

Head & Neck Region:
No abnormal soft tissue mass or FDG uptake is evident in the tonsil, thyroid, pharynx, nasopharynx or larynx. The visualised portions of the para-nasal sinuses are clear.

Skeleton:
No hypermetabolic sclerotic or lytic destruction is identified. No abnormal FDG accumulation is observed in the marrow to suggest bone metastasis. There is no pathological fracture or vertebral collapse seen. Minor spinal spondylitic changes are evident.

COMMENT:
Status CA right lung post VATS and chemotherapy, with mets in brain, nodes and Rt pleura.

The current study shows good treatment response.

The activities of the mediastinal nodal and right pleural diseases have decreased with some nodes are resolved. The Rt SCF node is resolved.

The right sided pleural effusion has diminished. The RLL atelectasis is stable and hypometabolic.

No brain metastasis is discernible.

No new metastasis is detected at the adrenals, liver, left hemithorax & bones.

MBBS (HK), FRCR (UK), FHKCR, FHKAM (Radiology)

Patient Name	: CHAN		
Sex/Age	: M/ 59	Examination Date	: 12/11/2010
		Reported Date	: 12/11/2010
Examination	: WHOLE BODY PET CT SCAN		

CT. Brain With IV contrast:
There is no abnormal density or contrast enhancement is detected in the leptomeninges, cerebral or cerebellar hemispheres. No cerebral oedema is seen. There is no deviation of the midline structure.

The ventricles are of normal dimensions. Normal sulcal and gyral pattern is present over both cerebral hemispheres. The pituitary gland and pineal gland are not enlarged. The brainstem and cerebellum are normally defined.

No extra-dural collection or calvarial destruction is observed.

COMMENT: No new deposit has developed in the brain.

Whole Body PET-CT Scan:
This is a follow-up study; the current findings are compared with last study 08/2010.

Thorax (table 1):
There have been previous VATS at the right lung.

There is no evidence of abnormal metabolism to suggest local recurrence at the surgical site and right lung.

The right basal pleural effusion has diminished to 4.3cm (it was at 8.9cm) (image 101).

The focal atelectasis at the RLL basal segment remains stable (image 83) at 3.7 x 2.6cm, with FDG-uptake at SUVmax 1.9 (was at SUVmax 2.1).

The right pleural deposit has mild FDG-uptake at the postero-lateral aspect at SUVmax 2.

The calcified granulomata at the right and left lung apices are unchanged.

There is no pericardial effusion observed.

Node (table 1):
The multiple nodal deposits in the mediastinum have mild activities detected. The hottest node is now at SUVmax 2.9 (it was at SUVmax 6.3). The size is smaller with some is resolved. The right SCF node is also resolved. Please see table 1 for comparison.

No new hypermetabolic node is found at the neck, abdomen and pelvis.

Abdomen & Pelvis:
Both adrenals are not enlarged. No abnormal FDG-uptake is present in the adrenals.

No ascites or peritoneal deposit is found.

病案 4
没做化疗和放疗

曾先生是台湾的企业家,公司经营得很成功,他的电子产品畅销全国。2007年,他五十六岁,风华正茂,事业也处在巅峰,虽然亲朋都对他投以羡慕的眼光,但他知道,在成功的背后往往有比别人更多的付出,有的以后可补回来,有的则一去不返。

像是在跟时间竞赛,曾先生每天都马不停蹄地工作,经常往返全国各地,时常忘了进餐和休息。他的事业随着每天的努力步步高升,原以为这样下去,可登上人生的下一个高峰。但在2007年底,他感到精神不够、疲劳、体重不断下降、体力大不如前,在家人的关心及催促下,他终于下定决心去做身体检查。等待结果期间,他从没有想过自己会有什么大病,以为只是日夜奔波,才使他感觉疲惫不堪,只要多休息便可复原。但事实是残酷的,检查结果指出他患上了肺癌,而且肿瘤生长得很快。

服用中药后情况好转

在2008年1月,曾先生做了肺叶切除手术,之后医生又建议他做放疗和化疗，但经过多番了解，他明白这会带来很多不良反应。更令人担心的是，就算完成治疗亦有很大机会复发和转移，因此，他在与家人再三商讨后，最终决定不做放疗及化疗。他的家人在网上查阅各种治疗癌症的资料后，选择让他在术后3个月时到香港寻求中医药治疗。他初次求诊时身体状态很差，症见胸口疼痛、头痛、长期失眠、气促、多痰、呼吸困难，舌淡红，苔白腻，脉弦数，癌指数不断升高……病情非常严重！

治则：化湿祛毒，消癌散结。

常用中药：苍术、杏仁、海浮石、青礞石、生薏苡仁、干蟾皮、半夏、胆南星、瓜蒌、海藻、昆布，消瘤粉同时服用。

生薏苡仁，味甘，气香，入足太阴脾经、足阳明胃经。燥土清金，利水泻湿，善开胸痹，虽是一味平淡无奇的药，但能清能燥，兼利兼泻，具抑阴扶阳、祛浊化湿之力。苍术、杏仁助薏苡仁燥湿、止咳，海浮石、青礞石，化痰软坚，蟾皮利水、解毒。

患者脾虚痰湿，痰瘀互结，故以健脾化痰，解毒散结为主。经过抗癌中医药治疗，曾先生逐渐好转，体力亦慢慢加强，在从未做放疗及化疗的情况下身体状况依然良好。现在的他，对中医药深信不疑，亦有恒心地每天服药。五六年过去了，曾先生跟没患肺癌前一样，奔波于全国各地。十五年过去了，他仍然精力充沛，工作投入，现在还经常前来用生命修复法调理身体。

同期患癌朋友不治

前些日子，他来香港就诊时，讲述了两件事，这两件事使他对生命修复抗癌中医药治疗充满信心。一件事是当年他刚发现有癌症时，他的主诊医生，一位六十岁左右姓李的医生，是台湾大学医学院附设医院胸腔外科主任，也是专门医治肺癌的。这位医生后来也患上了肺癌，只是这位癌症专家从发现癌症到过世，只有几个月而已，曾先生深信这位医生会使用最先进和最现代化的西医治癌手段为自己治疗。

另一件事是他同事，五十多岁，与他年龄相仿，发现患肺癌的时间也相近。当时这位朋友打电话给他，告诉他很抱歉不能来看望他，因为自己也验出有肺癌，正在进一步治疗。之后他接受手术及化疗，但6个月后不幸复发，再做化疗，半年后不治去世。

透过自身及身边朋友的经历，曾先生感慨万千，庆幸自己多年来选择了合适的治疗方法，从而重获生命。

病案 5
把握阴阳调平衡，肺癌已度十八年

1999年魏女士身处美国，因为咳嗽、胸痛而发现肺部肿瘤，医生抽取肺组织做病理检查之后，确诊为肺癌。

同年8月，魏女士在美国进行了手术，切除了整个左上肺叶以及左下肺叶的两个肿瘤。然而这种肺内有扩散、转移性癌肿的情况是很严重的，且属于癌症晚期，即使做了切除手术，复发的可能性仍非常高。所以，美国的医生决定每六个月就为她做一次检查，以便能够及时发现新的问题并做适当处理。

术后不足三年两肺现四肿瘤

果然不出院方所料，在2002年6月，在魏女士例行的磁共振、CT扫描检查中发现两肺共有四个新的肿瘤出现。

魏女士当时在香港，当她得知肿瘤复发后，立即打电话找她的医生详细询问，希望能够再回到美国做进一步治疗。美国的医生对她的病况很了解，虽然美国有更加先进的医疗技术，但这种术后肿瘤复发的病况是很严重的，实际上也没有有效的治疗方法，即便再返回美国治疗，医生心中也并无把握。

魏女士在电话中询问了很久也没有得到肯定的回答。她只好试探问问，用中医药治疗可以吗？美国那边的医生正左右为难，虽然并不了解中医药，但在没有更好办法的情况下，未尝不可将中医药作为一种新的治疗方法试试，所以赞同她试用中医药治疗。魏女士于是来寻求生命修复抗癌中医药治疗，开始服用中药。

来诊时她全身疲乏无力，精神差、失眠、气促、胸闷、腰膝酸软、尿频失禁、呼吸不能连续，每说一句话，即需要大力换一口气。

治则：补肾培元，祛邪攻癌。

常用中药：熟地黄、百合、蛤蚧、半夏、杏仁、苏子、木鳖子、炙甘草、麦冬、肉苁蓉。

熟地黄、蛤蚧补益肺肾，麦冬、柏子仁、炙甘草益心肺，半夏、杏仁、苏子、木鳖子化瘀降逆抗癌。软坚散同服。

患者年老，正气不足，癌毒元盛，吸气少，呼气多，心气不足，肾不纳气均有。

魏女士认真遵照医嘱服用中药，呼吸困难等症逐渐缓解，病情逐渐好转。在用抗癌中医药治疗半年后，即2002年12月，再做CT检查，结果显示已恢复正常。患者对治疗效果非常满意，现在没有任何肿瘤复发的迹象。当然提供报告的放射科医生并不知道这个非常满意的治疗效果是来自中医药的。

自魏女士患肺癌至今，寒来暑往，已有十八个年头。她照样每年做检查，结果都证实肺癌没有再复发。

苦药换健康，旅行体验人生

这些年来，她一直用中药调理身体。前几年，她有时会抱怨中药的味道苦，感到服食苦药不舒服。在医生的开导下，她对这件事有了新的看法。她想，暂时服用一点苦药能换来身体的健康是很值得的。况且，人的口感、味觉也需要常常调整，总是香甜的味道也不见得是好事，从中医理论来讲，辛、甘、酸、苦、咸不同的味道，对人的身体是有不同的作用和影响的，均衡并常调整才更为科学。魏女士的抗癌中医药治疗原则是调理阴阳失衡，益气培元，散结解毒。肺为华盖，长期治疗以顾护正气为先。如今魏女士已有七十多岁了，她精神良好，生活质量很高，经常到世界各地旅游，寻求开心和体验人生。

肺癌是当今最难治、发病率和死亡率最高的恶性肿瘤之一。魏女士虽经肺叶手术切除，仍无法避免复发，千千万万这样复发后的患者，在再次经过短时间的化疗或放疗后，仍不能延续生命。魏女士没采用化疗、放疗，而选择用了抗癌中医药治疗，如今已有十八年了，她生活正常，身体健康。

诊疗记录

魏女士，61岁，肺癌手术后复发转移。

1999年11月8日手术后检查报告证实为肺腺癌。

2002年6月18日MRI/CT/SCAN报告两肺发现有4个新的病灶，他们分别位于：①右肺下叶；②左肺底；③右肺底；④左肺上叶。

2002年12月7日CT，SCAN，报告与3个月前检查比较，治疗反应良好，在肺部、纵隔、肺门、胸膜、胸骨等部位均没有见到有任何肿瘤复发。

2007年1月6日CT，SCAN再次检查报告：全身器官均正常。

2012年2月24日再次检查报告正常。

附：患者检查报告

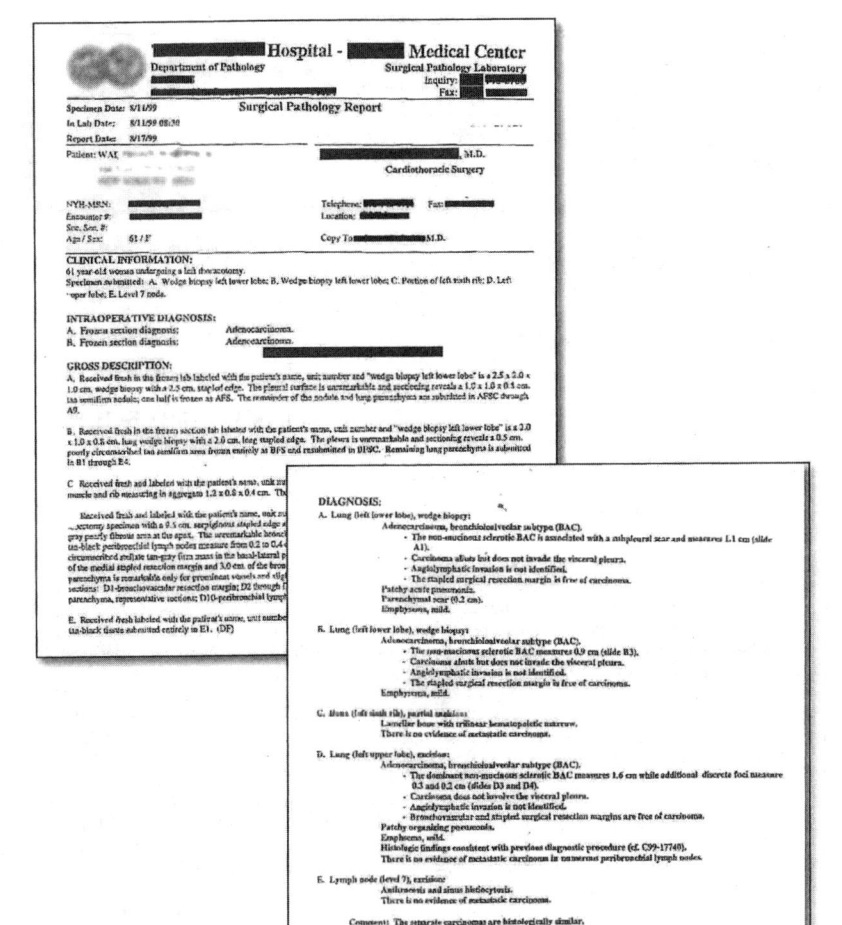

HOSPITAL
SCANNING DEPARTMENT
(CT, MR, NM, Mammography, U/S, Bone Densitometry)

Tel.:

REPORT FOR MRI/CT/NM SCANNING EXAMINATION

NAME	: CT ▇▇ 02		EXAM. DATE	: Tue, 18 Jun. 2002
ID No.	: B24			
AGE / SEX	: 64 F		HOSPITAL	: OUT-PATIENT
DATE	: Tue, 18 Jun. 2002			
EXAM.	: CT of Thorax			

CONTRAST MEDIUM : Iopamiro 370   REF. DR. :

CLINICAL HISTORY:

Bronchioalveolar cell carcinoma for follow-up. Small meningioma in brain, definite, not a metastasis also for follow-up.

RADIOLOGICAL REPORT:

5 mm collimation high resolution axial helical scans have been performed with and without contrast injection. One set of non-contrast images from the previous examination on 1 December, 2001 is also printed for comparison. A minute 2 mm nodule is shown in the anterior aspect of the right lower lung field is again shown (page 4, image 39). This lesion was present in previous examination also image 39. Previous opinion was said it is benign and this is a correct diagnosis. In the meantime the lesion has not increase in size at all.

There are total of four new lesions identifiable. One is located in the antero-medial aspect of the right lower lung about 2.5 cm above the level of the 2 mm lesion and shown in image 34. Its size is 26 x 19 mm along the transaxial plane. It is immediately subpleural in location and close to midline. Prior to contrast injection, density measurement ranging from 5 to 20. After contrast injection, there is enhancement ranging from 15 units to 40 units. A second lesion is shown in the shape of a fan and it is quite small in size measuring no more than 2 cm in diameter and is located in the posterior portion of the left lung base (image 47). It did not exist in previous examination. A third lesion is noted in the posterior right lung base. It is quite hazy in character and poorly defined in the boundaries. 1 mm images show the same characteristics. It may well be an area of pneumonitis and so is the second lesion. A fourth lesion is shown which is of the same hazy character and located in the postero-medial aspect of the left upper lung.

Post-contrast scan shows no sign of any mediastinal or hilar lymphadenopathy. Regional bones show no metastatic disease.

Hospital

Scanning Department
(CT, MR, NM, PET Scan, Bone Densitometry)

REPORT FOR MRI/CT/NM/PET SCANNING EXAMINATION

OUR REF. : CT ▬▬▬ 02	EXAM. DATE :	Sat, 7 Dec, 2002
NAME : Wai ▬▬▬		
ID No. : B24▬▬		
AGE / SEX : 64 F	HOSPITAL :	OUT-PATIENT
DATE : Mon, 9 Dec, 2002		
XAM. : CT of Thorax		
	REF. DR. :	▬▬▬▬▬
CONTRAST MEDIUM : Iopamiro 370		

CLINICAL HISTORY:

Bronchio-alveolar cell tumour, treated, for sequential follow-up.

RADIOLOGICAL REPORT:

Helical scan has been performed with high resolution technique. Left upper lung field shows linear densities representing scars both in the peripheral lung and in the perihilar region. Comparison with previous examination indicates that all the shadows existing in the lungs were previously presented including the small nodule in the anterior aspect of the right lung base (image 44) which has not been enlarging at all with the passage of time. Post-contrast scan demonstrates that the different major areas of the mediastinum are also normal without enlarged lymph node while the regional bones including the thoracic spine show no sign of plastic or lytic lesion.

OPINION :

This post-treatment follow-up study is quite satisfactory. Last examination was done exactly 3 months ago in 7th Sept. 2002. No change is observed and there is no sign of any recurrence of tumour in the lungs, mediastinum, hilum, pleural space, regional bones or chest wall.

NO. OF FILMS : 9 14" x 17"

SIGNED
DR. ▬▬▬▬▬

治癌实录 2
中晚期癌症 · 名家手记

Hospital
Scanning Department
(CT, MR, NM, PET Scan, Bone Densitometry)

CT S........7
EXAM. DATE 6 Jan, 2007

REPORT FOR MRI/CT/NM/PET SCANNING EXAMINATION

NAME Wai ███ ███ ███

ID No. B24█████   AGE 68   SEX F

ABDOMEN-

Study of the abdomen demonstrates once again large sized benign renal cyst in the upper part of the left kidney and the size of the cyst remains unchanged. Other abdominal organs are normal. In particular, the pancreas shows no pancreatitis or tumour mass. The lumen of the stomach is normal without any intrinsic lesion shown. Liver shows no nodular lesion and retroperitoneum as well as porta hepatis show no enlarged lymph node.

Opinion:

Benign left renal cyst is again noted and the size has not increased. Other abdominal organs are also quite normal.

SIGNED
DR.

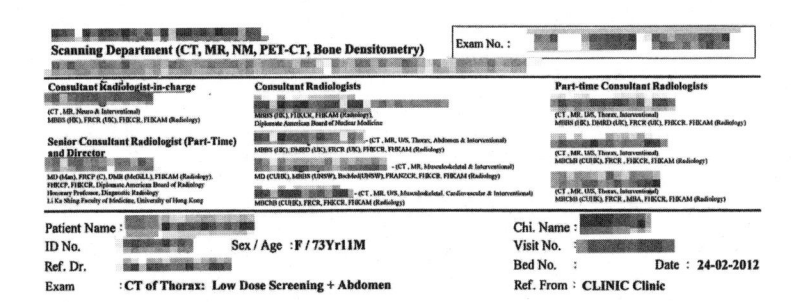

Scanning Department (CT, MR, NM, PET-CT, Bone Densitometry)	Exam No. :	

Consultant Radiologist-in-charge

Consultant Radiologists

Part-time Consultant Radiologists

Senior Consultant Radiologist (Part-Time) and Director

Patient Name :		Chi. Name :	
ID No.	Sex / Age : F / 73Yr11M	Visit No. :	
Ref. Dr.		Bed No. :	Date : 24-02-2012
Exam	: CT of Thorax: Low Dose Screening + Abdomen	Ref. From : CLINIC Clinic	

Clinical Information / History:

History of alveolar cell carcinoma of lung. Follow-up for more than 5 years (in fact 13 years) and considered cured.
Previous examination showed left renal cysts and left adrenal adenoma. Patient would like to have general survey of abdominal organs.

Radiological Report:

THORAX (LOW DOSE SCREENING)-

High resolution low dose screening technique is applied. Linear scar exists in the anterior aspect of the left apex. Anterior aspect of left upper lung also contains calcification site as well as localized pleural thickening. No nodule or mass or consolidation or collapse or cavitory lesion is found in the lungs. Gross tortuosity of brachiocephalic vessels are shown bulging into the antero-medial aspect of the right apex, not to be mistaken for significant lung lesion. As far as I can see in this non-contrast CT scan, the mediastinum is unremarkable. Chest wall, axilla and supraclavicular region show no pathology to note.

Opinion:

There is no sign of recurrence of malignancy in the thorax.

病案 6
治九旬长者食管癌

人口老龄化,是世界各发达国家需要共同面对的挑战。社会变迁,老年人口不断增加,癌症及慢性病的发病率越来越高,随之而来的死亡率也逐渐增加。

老年人癌症发病率较高,常见癌症包括乳腺癌、膀胱癌、直肠癌、肺癌及肝癌等。老年人除了发病率高,确诊时亦多属晚期,患者往往出现严重消瘦、不能进食、食欲差、疲倦、水肿、呕吐、失眠、头痛及大小便困难等症状。

老年癌症患者还容易出现淋巴转移、肿瘤压迫引起疼痛、水肿、骨转移引起骨疼痛等,而且他们的癌细胞更容易转移到其他器官。针对这些特殊情况,中医药在治疗老年人的癌症方面是有优势的。

多属晚期不适宜手术

老年人患癌症的比例也非常高,统计显示有三成多患癌老人,承受癌症所带来的痛症超过六个月以上。治疗老年癌症患者,应考虑到他们的特点做出针对性治疗。第一个特点是老年人常有非肿瘤的并发症,例如多数同时患有骨质增生、慢性腰腿疼痛、骨质疏松、骨关节炎、糖尿病、神经性疼痛、中风后遗症、排尿问题、尿道结石、胆石症、慢性胃病、慢性消化性问题及高血压等,并非单纯只有肿瘤;第二个特点是老年人通常身体较弱,免疫功能和抵抗能力都较差,加上癌症发现的时候往往都已是晚期,大多数都不宜接受手术,更不宜接受攻击性治疗。

老年癌症患者除了经常出现并发症外,身体承受能力也较差,往往难以承受手术、放疗及化疗的打击。例如统计显示,九成多食管癌的老年患者承受不了手术,而化疗与放疗的治疗效果也不理想。

黄老太93岁了,她于2012年初因吞咽困难、不能进食去医院就诊,被确诊为食管癌晚期并伴有肝转移。最初黄老太在医院接受了几次放疗,但很快就发现身体难以承受,全身状况迅速变差。医生指其生命随时可能出现危险,故放弃治疗。于是她来寻求抗癌中医药治疗。黄老太最初求诊时,身体严重消瘦、恶病质、不能进食、不能吞咽,仅食极少量流质,咽喉有大量痰液堵塞、大便数日不行、四肢不温,舌淡苔白,脉沉细,生命垂危。

治则：健运中焦，散结除癥。

常用中药：人参、干姜、砂仁、茯苓、鸡内金、半夏、黄药子、水红花子、牡蛎、竹茹、枳壳、大黄。

患者年老体弱，正气虚弱，邪气亢盛，阳衰土湿，上下之窍均闭阻，治疗必先顾及中焦脾胃，健运中焦则可开通上下之窍，进一步才可祛痰散结，下气通滞。人参、干姜、砂仁、茯苓为健运中焦的主药，半夏、黄药子、鸡内金，牡蛎均用以降逆、散结消积，半夏、竹茹、枳壳、大黄祛痰降逆，散结通滞。

老妇吞咽改善渐好转

黄老太在用抗癌中医药治疗后，吞咽逐渐改善，能进食较多流质，一个月后可以吃些饭；三个月后可进食固体食物，吃饭正常，每餐可进食一至两碗饭，精神、生活也都有明显好转。至 2012 年底，她到医院做例行检查，医护人员都感到很惊讶，没想到还能见到她。现在一年多过去，黄老太仍在接受抗癌中医药治疗，身体状态良好。黄老太愉快、平静地生活到 2015 年，以 96 岁高龄辞世，尽享天伦。

目前普遍认为，治疗老年的食管癌患者十分困难。随着社会人口老龄化，老年食管癌的发病率又越来越高。西医治疗食管癌的手术对身体会造成很大的创伤,然而这样的重大创伤,很多老年人都承受不了,就算完成手术,继后的化疗与放疗造成的伤害同样令患者承受不了,更莫说是年老长者;而且化疗及放疗会带来很多的不良反应,在此情况下,选用抗癌中医药治疗是比较好的。黄老太用中医药治疗食管癌,取得明显的效果,就是一个很好例子。

诊疗记录

2012年4月24日食管下部组织病理报告证实食管有恶性肿瘤。

2012年5月21日证实有胃及食管肿瘤并怀疑有肝转移。

2014年5月,黄女士复诊,身体状况良好。

治癌实录 2
中晚期癌症·名家手记

附：患者检查报告

A

URGENT

Lab No.:

Name: WONG.
MRN:

Sex/Age: F/91Y
Unit: PYN/SOP
Ref.:

Bed:

Date Collected: 24/04/12
Date Arrived: 24/04/12
Specimen: Esophagus

Final Report

Diagnosis :
ESOPHAGUS, OGJ tumour, biopsy :
- Compatible with ADENOCARCINOMA

Clinical data :
Epigastric mass
Suspected Cancer of oesophagus - thoracic lower third (530.9)

Gross Description :
OGJ tumour
4 pieces, 2 mm. All-embedded 1 block.

Microscopic description :
Section shows several pieces of mucosa at the squamo-columnar junction and glandular mucosa in papillary fragments. There is invasive abortive glands or tumour nests with stromal invasion. The tumour cells show moderate to marked pleomorphism and readily seen mitosis. High grade dysplasia is seen in the overlying glandular epithelium. No dysplasia is identified in the squamous epithelium.

The overall features are compatible with adenocarcinoma.

Final Report   18:26 on 25/04/12
                    ********** End of report **********

Report Destination:

* Screen capture report   Page 1
Printed on : 04/10/2012 15:40:45

A

放射科 **Department of Radiology** 檢驗報告 Examination Report	Case No.: HKID: Name: WONG, (黃　) Sex: F　　Age: 91y　　DOB: 01/01/1921

Imaging No.:　　　　　　　　　　　　　　　　　　　Exam Date : 21/05/2012 15:04

* DUPLICATE *

Examinations: Thorax plain, Thorax+con.,
Abdomen plain,...(More)

Contrast:
Iopamiro 370 100ml /bot 70.00 ml

Report:
Clinical History
adenoCA OGJ. for staging

Clinical Diagnosis
(SUR) Dysphagia
(SUR) Suspected Cancer of oesophagus - thoracic lower third (530.9)

(The above information has been automatically carried forward from referring clinician's GCRS entry.)

CT THORAX AND ABDOMEN (CONTRAST) :

PROTOCOL:
Plain and contrast enhanced portal venous phase axial scans performed through thorax and abdomen.

FINDING:
Pleural thickening and small subpleural nodules are seen in bilateral lung apices suggestive of old inflammatory change.

A 3 mm calcific granuloma is seen at the left upper lobe.

A 3 mm soft tissue nodule is seen in the periphery of the right lobe, another 3 mm soft tissue nodule is seen at periphery of right middle lobe. They are too small to be exactly characterized by CT, granulomas versus metastases. No enlarged mediastinal or hilar lymph nodes seen. No pleural effusion is detected.

A lobulated soft tissue mass, measuring approximately 40X32x25 mm (LSxAPxTS) is seen at the gastric fundus, in keeping with the known carcinoma. There is some suspicious extension into the lower oesophagus at the region of the hiatus. No conclusive infiltration into the perigastric fat is seen. A shotty perigastric lymph node measuring 5.6x8.1mm is seen. No enlarged celiac nor SMA lymph nodes seen.

Multiple hypo dense hypo enhancing lesions(some containing some small calcific foci) are seen in both lobes of the liver, largest 21x20 mm in the right lobe, suspicious of liver metastases.
Several well-defined cysts are also seen the liver.

A 22x23 mm hypodense lesion with rim calcification is seen in segment 6 right lobe of liver. A smaller lesion measuring 9.0x15 mm is seen lateral segment 3 left lobe. These are suggestive of old insult or inflammation, including hydatid cysts.

A 3 mm hypo enhancing lesion is noted at the lateral subcapsular region of the spleen, too small to be

Reported by :　　　　　　　　　　　on 21/05/2012 18:50

Printed on　:　04/10/2012 15:40

治癌实录 2

中晚期癌症・名家手记

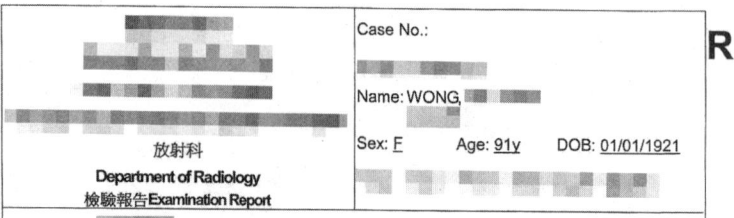

	Case No.:
放射科 **Department of Radiology** 檢驗報告 Examination Report	Name: WONG, Sex: F　Age: 91y　DOB: 01/01/1921

Imaging No.: 　　　　　　　　　　　　　　　　　　Exam Date : 21/05/2012 15:04

R
C
T

* *DUPLICATE* *

exactly characterized by CT.

No biliary tract dilatation is seen.
The gallbladder wall is not thickened with no stone or pericholecystic fluid.

The adrenals are not enlarged.

No conspicuous pancreatic mass detected. The pancreatic duct is prominent up to 3.5 mm, may represent atrophic change.

No renal mass or hydronephrosis detected. Several cortical cysts are seen, largest 5.3 cm at lower pole right kidney.

No ascites is seen in the upper abdomen.

Scoliosis of the upper lumbar spine convex to write is seen. Compression deformity of the T12 vertebral body is noted with height diminished by about 50%.

IMPRESSION :
1.Known carcinoma of the gastric fundus, with suspicious extension into the lower oesophagus at the region of the hiatus. No conclusive perigastric fat infiltration noted. Shotty perigastric lymph node is seen. Suspicious bilobed liver metastases. Non-specific tiny nodule at right upper and right middle lobe and at periphery of the spleen.
2. Other findings as above.

on 21/05/2012 18:50

Printed on　:　04/10/2012 15:40

Page 2 of 2

病案 7
补中消瘤，转危为安

钟女士（73岁）2006年确诊胃癌，接受手术切除了大半边胃，手术时发现已有淋巴转移，并可能伴有肝转移，手术后医生又安排了化疗和放疗。她说记得那时每日都要去医院做化疗和放疗，非常痛苦，但终于还是熬过了这段相当长的艰难岁月。

没想到好景不长，术后仅三年，即2009年，钟女士因腹痛去医院检查，又发现了肠癌。医生说这是一个新肿瘤，并非转移来的，需要再次安排手术切除。别人患一种癌症已非常严重，钟女士竟然患了两种癌，她和家人都感到很可怕。

两次手术减了20磅

钟女士很想知道她为什么这样不幸，为什么会患上两种癌症。经过多方了解和查阅书籍，他们终于明白化疗和放疗本身都有化学和放射毒害，本身就有导致癌症发生的可能。她在胃癌术后长久地化疗和放疗，就很有可能导致第二种癌症的发生。

钟女士又按照医生的要求，决定尽快再次做手术切除肠癌，就在即将做手术之前又有麻烦发生。她因为感染出现了急性肾衰竭，需要先洗肾才能够做手术。

首次手术以后，钟女士的体重减了10磅；第二次手术后，再减轻了10磅，这使她虚弱不堪，与之前判若两人，亲朋好友见到她都不敢相认。她自己也感到生命快到尽头。术后肾功能继续转差，癌指数却不断上升，肾功能更出现衰竭，无法再接受化疗。

在没有其他办法下，钟女士转用抗癌中医药治疗。初诊时她的身体极度虚弱，由于呕吐、胀满，连中药也无法吞咽，只有安排抗癌及固本同时进行少量多次地煎煮服用中药。来诊时见胸闷腹胀、嗳气频作、脘腹胀痛、时时呕吐、大便不畅，舌淡苔白，脉沉弦。

治则：通腑泄毒，通滞消瘤。

常用中药：党参、白术、山药、厚朴、大黄、芦荟、鸡内金、土鳖虫、地榆、槟榔、高良姜、半夏、柴胡、香附。消瘤粉、散结丸同时服用。

六腑以通为用，患者胃腑肠道都出现恶性肿瘤，应行气化痰、通下。大黄、芦荟、厚朴、槟榔、地榆均为通腑泄毒的常用药，患者年老体弱，要同时顾及中气，故用党参、白术、山药等补药。鸡内金、土鳖虫、槟榔、香附等，行气通滞止痛、化瘀消瘤。

除了患有胃癌、肠癌及发生转移外，钟女士还有高血压、肾衰竭、腹痛、失眠、咳嗽、头晕、疲乏无力等症，全部要靠抗癌中医药治疗。当时医院就曾告诉她，因为她不能化疗，很快就会发生肺和肝的转移，生命已非常危险。

计算一下，从患癌症至今，已11年过去了。她坚持服用中药，身体良好，已没有任何不适。每次来看病时，问她有什么不舒服，她总是回答："什么都没有，能吃能睡，生活完全正常。"自从采用抗癌中医药治疗后，钟女士身体状况良好，血压正常、肾功能正常，也没有发生医院里早就预言过的全身多脏器癌症转移及复发的情况。

很有意思的是，钟女士回想起几个月前去医院进行常规的检查，香港的一位西医在看完她的血液检查显示肾功能等指标在正常范围以及肿瘤并没有复发的事实后，告诉她说："现在情况良好，你保持这样很不简单呀，可定期来做检查，但千万不要吃中药，否则就会迅速恶化。"钟女士没有回应他。但她说，如果没有生命修复抗癌中医治疗，她早已没有命了。

诊疗记录

2006年10月20日CT报告证实患溃疡性胃癌,怀疑肝转移。

2006年10月31日病理报告证实为胃低分化腺癌。

2009年7月30日病理报告证实患浸润性肠腺癌,淋巴转移。

2017年2月5日随访,钟女士生活正常。

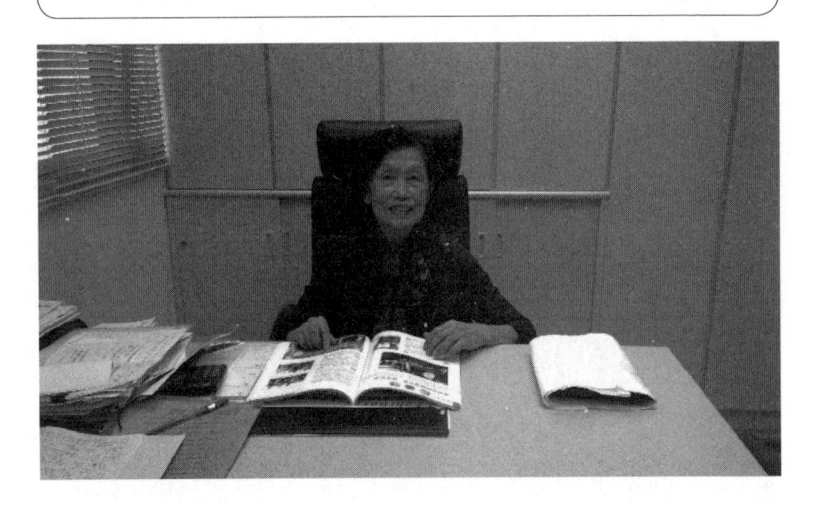

附：患者检查报告

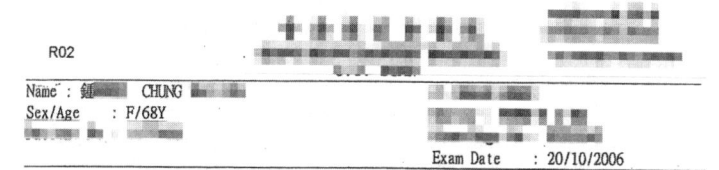

R02

Name : 鍾 CHUNG
Sex/Age : F/68Y

Exam Date : 20/10/2006

Exam : WHOLE ABDOMEN (P + C)

REPORT :

There is an ulcer crater with enhancing mucosal thickening demonstrated in the gastric pylorus which likely represents the biopsy proven malignant gastric ulcer. It measures about 1.56cm x 2.45cm x 4.93cm in size. There is associated nonspecific gastric wall thickening extending into the distal pyloric antrum. No gross extra-luminal tumour infiltration of the perigastric fat or adjacent structure demonstrated. No significant regional enlarged lymphadenopathy demonstrated.

There are two nonspecific small nodules in the left lung base (0.42cm and 0.25cm). No discrete focal lesion identified in the right lung base. No pleural effusion demonstrated.

No gross erosive bone lesion demonstrated. Small sclerotic foci in the pelvic girdle may represent small bone islands.

There are multiple well-defined hypodense hypoenhancing foci in both lobes of liver which may represent hepatic cysts, although cystic metastases from adenocarcinoma cannot be definitely excluded, the largest in the left lobe measures 1.66cm x 2.07cm x 1.54cm and the largest in the right lobe measures 1.08cm x 1.72cm x 1.63cm. No gross biliary ductal dilatation demonstrated. The portal veins, hepatic veins and IVC are patent. The gallbladder appears normal, no hyperdense gallstone demonstrated.

The pancreas is normal in size and configuration with normal homogeneous enhancement. The pancreatic duct is not dilated. The spleen is not enlarged. No gross adrenal mass lesion demonstrated.

Both kidneys are normal in size, position and axis of alignment. Smooth renal contour with no evidence of renal scarring. Preserved renal cortical thickness on both sides. No hyperdense urolithiasis or

C T S C A N

Date: 20/10/2006 16:56   Page: 1 of 3   /cy
C.T. SCAN

R02

Name : 鍾 ░░ CHUNG ░░ ░░
Sex/Age : F/68Y

Exam Regn No : ░░
Exam Date : 20/10/2006

hydroureteronephrosis demonstrated. Both kidneys show normal enhancement and contrast excretion. Tiny renal cysts noted in both kidneys.

Normal abdominal aortic calibre. No significant enlarged para-aortic, iliac or mesenteric lymphadenopathy demonstrated. No significant ascites demonstrated. No sign of pneumoperitoneum.

No gross small bowel or large bowel mass lesion demonstrated. The appendix appears normal. No evidence of colonic diverticulosis/diverticulitis.

There are multiple calcified lesions in the uterus which likely represent calcified uterine leiomyomas, the largest measures 2.75cm x 2.42cm x 3.26cm. No pelvic/adnexal mass lesion demonstrated. No pelvic focal collection or significant free fluid shown. The bilateral ischiorectal fossae are clear.

CONCLUSION:

There is an ulcer crater with enhancing mucosal thickening demonstrated in the gastric pylorus which likely represents the biopsy proven malignant gastric ulcer. It measures about 1.56cm x 2.45cm x 4.93cm in size. There is associated nonspecific gastric wall thickening extending into the distal pyloric antrum. No gross extra-luminal tumour infiltration of the perigastric fat or adjacent structure demonstrated. No significant regional enlarged lymphadenopathy demonstrated.

There are multiple well-defined hypodense hypoenhancing foci in both lobes of liver which may represent hepatic cysts, although cystic metastases from adenocarcinoma cannot be definitely excluded, the largest in the left lobe measures 1.66cm x 2.07cm x 1.54cm and the largest in the right lobe measures 1.08cm x 1.72cm x 1.63cm.

There are two nonspecific small nodules in the left lung base. No discrete focal lesion identified in the right lung base. No pleural effusion demonstrated.

Date: 20/10/2006 16:56   Page: 2 of 3   /cy
C.T. SCAN

PATIENT'S NAME	DATE RECEIVED	PATHOLOGY NO.	COPY:
CHUNG	31/10/2006		DR. HOSP OTHERS
I.D .NO	SEX F	AGE 68 Y	
HOSPITAL	HOSPITAL NO.	CLASS	PREVIOUS PATH. NO.

UNDER CARE OF DR.

DOCTOR'S ADDRESS

CLINICAL PROCEDURE — Distal radical gastrectomy, excision common hepatic artery lymph node.

CLINICAL SUMMARY — CA stomach. S/P distal radical gastrectomy. Left gastric lymph node mark with stitch.

FROZEN SECTION DIAGNOSIS (If any) — Proximal margin - Benign.

PATHOLOGICAL DIAGNOSIS
(1) & (2) Stomach (distal radical gastrectomy)
- Poorly differentiated adenocarcinoma, T2bN0, completely excised.
(Pending immunohistochemistry)
(3) Common hepatic artery lymph node - Benign.
(Pending immunohistochemistry)

REPORT

Macroscopic examination:

(1) "Proximal margin" - A light-brown piece of tissue 3.2 x 1.4 x 0.7 cm.

(2) "Distal stomach" - Specimen consisted of distal stomach, lesser curve 11 cm. long, greater curve 14.2 cm. long, proximal margin 5 cm. in diameter, distal margin 1.5 cm. in diameter, cut-open before receipt. The serosal surfaces were indurated at the greater curve. 5.2 cm. from the distal margin was an ulcerated light-brown firm tumour 2.2 x 1.6 cm. in area, 0.2 cm. deep with necrotic base. Cut surfaces showed infiltration into thickened muscular wall (1.2 cm. thick), adjacent to the greater curve posteriorly. Greater omental fat measured 21 x 19.5 x 1.5 cm., lesser curve fat 9.3 x 3.7 x 1.4 cm. There were eight proximal lesser curve lymph nodes adjacent to the stitch on the lesser curve, largest 0.7 x 0.3 x 0.2 cm., smallest 0.2 cm. in diameter, and twelve distal greater curve lymph nodes, largest 1.2 x 0.8 x 0.4 cm. and smallest 0.2 cm. in diameter.

(3) "Common hepatic artery lymph node" - A brownish-yellow piece of tissue 2.1 x 1.3 x 0.4 cm. with four lymph nodes, largest 1.3 x 0.6 x 0.5 cm. and smallest 0.3 x 0.2 x 0.1 cm.

Microscopic examination:

(1) Paraffin section confirms the frozen section diagnosis and shows gastric mucosa without dysplasia or malignancy.

(PLEASE TURN OVERLEAF)

治癌实录 2
中晚期癌症・名家手记

PATIENT'S NAME	DATE RECEIVED	PATHOLOGY NO.	COPY:
CHUNG	31/10/2006		DR. HOSP OTHERS
I.D NO	SEX F	AGE 68 Y		
HOSPITAL	HOSPITAL NO	CLASS	PREVIOUS PATH NO	

UNDER CARE OF DR.

DOCTOR'S ADDRESS

CLINICAL PROCEDURE: Distal radical gastrectomy, excision common hepatic artery lymph node.

CLINICAL SUMMARY: CA stomach. S/P distal radical gastrectomy. Left gastric lymph node mark with stitch.

FROZEN SECTION DIAGNOSIS (if any): Proximal margin - Benign.

PATHOLOGICAL DIAGNOSIS:
Stomach (distal radical gastrectomy)
- Poorly differentiated adenocarcinoma, T2bN1, completely excised.
- 1/24 lymph nodes involved.

REPORT

Supplementary Report

Immunostaining for cytokeratin shows infiltration of one distal greater curve lymph node, not seen on superficial levels of the paraffin block. The other lymph nodes, including the common hepatic artery lymph nodes, are negative.

Date Reported: 04/11/2006

Signed: _____
MBBChir(Cantab), FRCPath(UK)
FHKCPath, FHKAM(Path)

Pathology Report

SPECIMEN TYPE
Right hemicolectomy.

CLINICAL DETAILS
Perforated appendiceal base + caecal tumour.

MACROSCOPIC EXAMINATION
Specimen received fresh and subsequently fixed in formalin with patient's data and designated colon. It consists of right colon, appendix and terminal ileum. The colonic segment measures 16 cm in length and 10 cm in maximum circumference at the caecum and 7 cm in maximum circumference at the ascending colon. The appendix measures 6 cm long and 1 cm in maximum diameter. The small intestine segment measures 35 cm long and 4 cm in maximum diameter. Outer surface of the colon, caecum and distal ileum is covered with inflammatory exudate. The appendix is dilated and covered with exudate. Small perforation is noted at the base of appendix. On opening, there is polypoid tan colored firm tumour at the caecum covering the appendiceal orifice, measuring 4 x 4 x 3 cm. It is 11 cm away from the distal resection margin and 35 cm from the proximal resection margin. The retro-caecal circumferential margin is inked blue, the perforation area is inked black and the rest of the serosal surface is inked yellow. Serial sections show whitish infiltrative tumour infiltrating the muscle coat and extending into the subserosal soft tissue, close to the perforation area. Multiple lymph nodes are identified in the mesenteric fat. The largest one measures 2 cm in maximum dimension. No soft tissue tumoral deposit is noted grossly.
Block 1 - proximal resection margin.
Block 2 - distal resection margin.
Block 3 - apical mesenteric resection margin.
Blocks 4 to 8 - tumour with the perforation area.
Block 9 - polypoid part of the tumour.
Block 10 - appendix.
Block 11 - circumferential margin (contain one lymph node bisected).
Blocks 12 to 14 - apical lymph nodes (blocks 13 and 14 - one lymph node bisected each).
Blocks 15 to 17 - caecal lymph nodes (block 17 - two lymph nodes, the largest is bisected).
Block 18 - lymph nodes of ascending colon.
Blocks 19 & 20 - ileal lymph nodes.
Block 21 - sampling of the small bowel.
Block 22 - sampling of the small bowel.
Block 23 - sampling of the caecum.

MICROSCOPIC EXAMINATION
Sections show a moderately differentiated adenocarcinoma forming cribriform and irregular angulated glandular pattern with focal mucin extravasation. The tumour shows moderate nuclear pleomorphism and hyperchromasia. Lympho-vascular permeation is not apparent. Adenomatous changes with low grade dysplasia is focally seen at the edge of the adenocarcinoma. Lymphoid reaction towards the tumor is mild. The tumor invades through

* Ward enquiry -- screen capture
Printed on : 12/08/2009 11:39:44

Page 1   to be continued...

治癌实录 2
中晚期癌症・名家手记

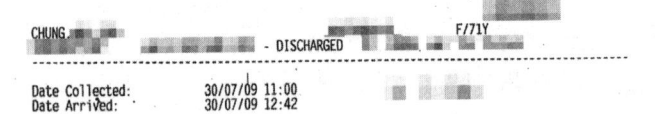

CHUNG   - DISCHARGED   F/71Y

Date Collected: 30/07/09 11:00
Date Arrived: 30/07/09 12:42

the muscularis propria. Serosa is not involved. Resection margins, including the apical mesenteric, circumferential, proximal and distal margins are clear. Two out of 14 paracolic lymph nodes show metastasis. The 10 apical and 9 ileal lymph nodes are negative for malignancy.
The perforation site at the base of appendix is noted and accompany with abscess formation and inflamed fibrosing granulation tissue. No malignant gland is seen at the perforation site. A sessile serrated adenoma is noted at the tip of appendix.

DIAGNOSIS
Right hemicolectomy:
-Moderately-differentiated Adenocarcinoma of cecum.
-Invades through muscularis propria.
-Serosa is not involved.
-Two out of 33 lymph nodes show metastasis.
-Resection margins are clear.
-pT3N1.
-Perforation at base of appendix with abscess and granulation tissue formation.
-Sessile serrated adenoma of appendix noted.

Pathology Report   Authorized By: 06/08/09 10:29
                    *** This Laboratory is NATA & RCPA accredited ***
                    ********** End of report **********

Report Destination:

病案 8
无毒无害治大病

手术、化疗及放疗是当前西医治癌的常用方法，但并不适用于所有癌症患者，尤其是年老的患者。年纪越大，手术风险就越高，化疗与放疗都有年龄和体质的限制。美国肿瘤协会 2001 年公布，不提倡 60 岁以上的恶性肿瘤患者接受化疗，因为年纪越大，身体的承受能力越低，而且化疗对正常细胞、免疫细胞都造成伤害。老年癌症患者再接受化疗或放疗等创伤性治疗方式，可谓雪上加霜，对患者的身体造成的打击更可能成为加速死亡的原因。

放疗与化疗本身，并无具备识别良、恶细胞的能力，也就是说"敌友不分"，治疗过程中往往同时灭杀体内大量的正常细胞，老年人往往难以承受这样攻击性的治疗。临床治疗过程中，经常有年老体弱的患者最终被迫终止放疗及化疗，这样不仅未能产生治疗作用，反而会令身体造成损伤甚至危及生命。

求助中医避手术

郑先生（86岁）一年前在家中突然中风昏倒，送入医院救治。入院两天后再次中风，左侧上下肢均瘫痪不能活动。检查后发现颈部大动脉有80%堵塞，而且还发生了急性脑梗死，需要立即行颈动脉血管手术和疏通血管等手术。但是在准备手术的过程中，郑先生又被查出患有晚期胃癌，因肿瘤很大，医院建议行全胃切除。

医院中两个不同的部门都要求尽快手术治疗，否则会有生命危险。家中儿女们方寸大乱，完全不知该怎么办。在焦虑无助下，儿女们决定将老人从医院接出来，先看看中医药有没有办法。经过几天治疗，患者病情逐渐稳定。他们再次考虑是否应当做手术，因患者年龄大，病情严重，身体又非常虚弱，两种手术都有很大的风险，所以最后家人一致决定放弃手术，用生命修复抗癌中医药治疗。症见神志模糊，左侧上下肢软瘫、麻木、喉中痰鸣、吞咽困难、腹部胀满、剑下压痛明显，舌暗苔白腻，脉左寸浮紧，右细沉。

治则：补正扶阳，消散瘀滞。

常用中药：制附子、丹参、地龙、石见穿、怀牛膝、路路通、桃仁、红花、苍术、生薏苡仁、藤梨根、九香虫。消瘤1号同时服用。

两侧脉极不平均，阴阳失衡。《黄帝内经》言"阴平阳秘，精神乃治，阴阳离决，精气乃绝"，左寸脉浮而紧，浮则为虚，紧则为寒。寒虚相搏，病发为中风，右脉细细，气滞日久，发为血瘀，经脉阻滞不行，清气不升，浊气不降，病情危重，治宜先用针灸，调整左右经脉之平衡，并艾灸关元，固肾益精，再用中药温补先天后天，通经化瘀，行滞消瘤，达到温肾，行气通滞的效果。

在以后的治疗中，郑先生肢体逐渐恢复活动，饮食也逐渐正常，精神好转，肿瘤逐渐缩小。他在三年中接受中医药的治疗，自己说，能吃能睡、精神好，已没有不适的感觉。

然而郑先生三年后在友人安排下又去医院接受西医治疗，因无法承受而去世。

药性温和适合长者

抗癌中医药治疗是一种可靠、安全、无毒副作用的治疗方法，注重全身的治理，明显较适合中晚期的老年癌症患者。抗癌中医药治疗的主要特点是方式温和，并能根据患者不同的疾病和体质特点，辨证施治，同时注重全身的调整治理，例如对老年人治疗多以治本为主，标本兼治，即便是完全不同系统的疾病也可以同期治疗。

例如郑先生患有脑梗死和胃癌，原来要做两个不同部位的手术，以86岁的高龄做两次这样的手术，风险极大。但中医药从整体出发，根据患者本身的状况辨证施治，全面调理，最终使患者免除了手术的极大风险和痛苦，也取得了良好的治疗效果。

诊疗记录

2012年5月2日CT报告证实患有胃癌，癌肿瘤在胃底部，并蔓延至胃、食管连接部位，淋巴转移。

2012年5月9日MRI证实郑先生患急性多发脑梗死，并有较陈旧的脑梗死、脑出血、严重颈动脉狭窄等。

2013年7月8日随访，郑先生生活正常。

抗癌治验录 下篇

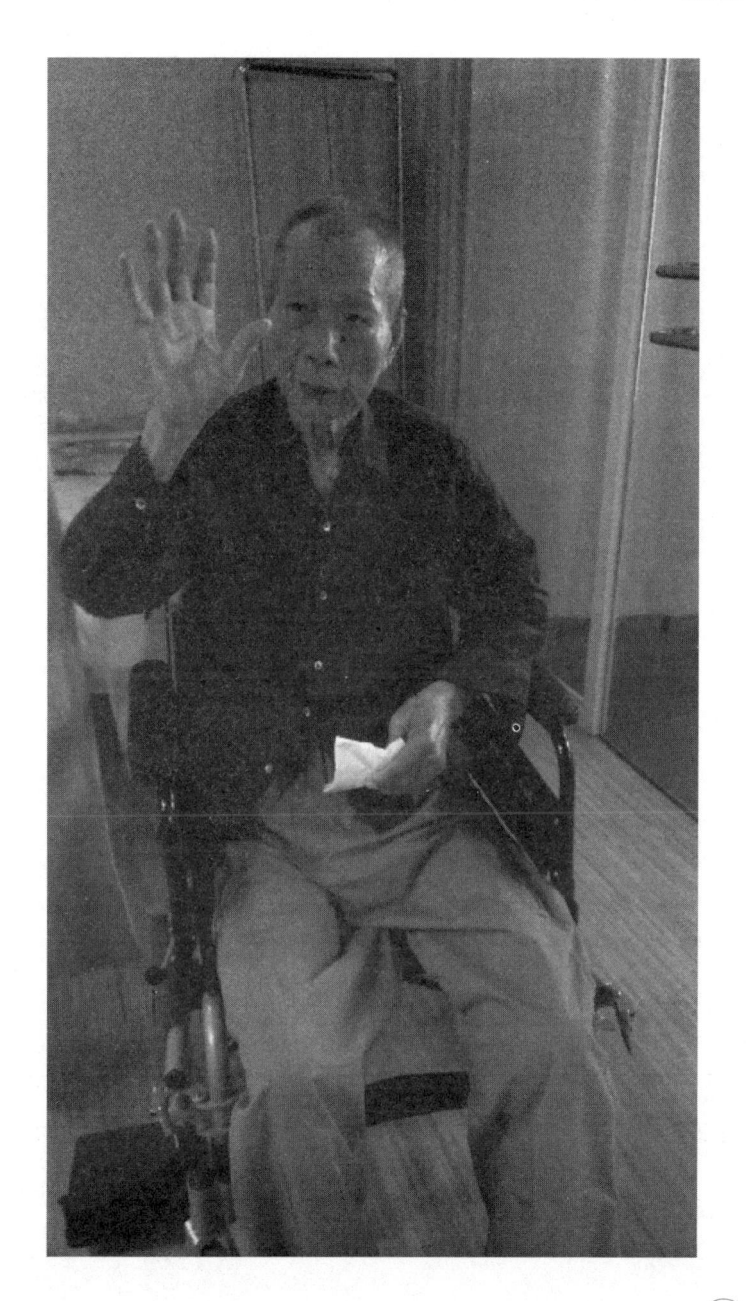

治癌实录 2

中晚期癌症·名家手记

附：患者检查报告

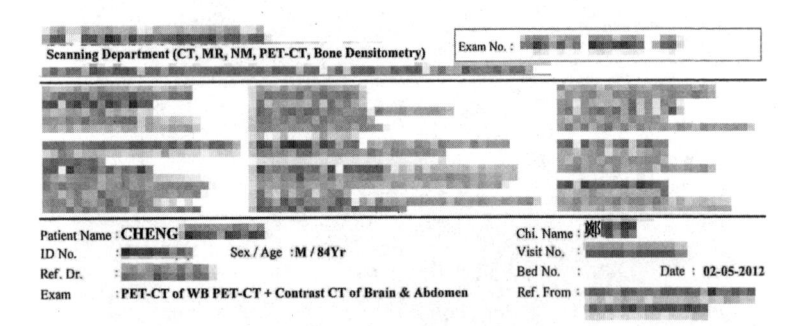

Scanning Department (CT, MR, NM, PET-CT, Bone Densitometry)

Exam No. :

Patient Name : CHENG		Chi. Name : 郑	
ID No. :	Sex / Age : M / 84Yr	Visit No. :	
Ref. Dr. :		Bed No. :	Date : 02-05-2012
Exam : PET-CT of WB PET-CT + Contrast CT of Brain & Abdomen		Ref. From :	

Comment:

Ill-defined hypodensity is seen involving the cortical region and subcortical region of the right parietal lobe with blurring of grey/white differentiation. The overlying cortex shows strong enhancement after contrast injection. No associated perifocal oedema or mass effect is seen. Hypodensity is also seen at the right basal ganglia and right internal capsule. No associated enhancement or mass effect is seen. Features are probably due to areas of recent infarct with luxurious perfusion at the lesion at the right parietal lobe. With the absence of enhancement at the right basal ganglia / internal capsular lesion, it is not typical of metastasis. Possibility of metastasis for the lesion at cortical region of right parietal lobe cannot be totally excluded and follow up CT or MR would be useful to monitor progress and ensures its benign nature if necessary. The rest of the brain is unremarkable. No midline shift is seen. No intracranial haemorrhage is noted. No abnormal extraaxial fluid collection is seen. Ventricular systems is not dilated. No regional bone erosion is seen.

CT ABDOMEN -

Techniques:

Pre-contrast helical axial scans of abdomen 10 mm.
Post-contrast helical axial scans of abdomen during portal phase 5 mm.
Multiplanar reformation.

Findings:

Enhancing wall thickening is seen along the upper part of lesser curve of stomach with involvement of the gastro-osephagyeal junction (SE 5 IM 19-22 film 9) consistent with carcinoma of stomach. The lesion measures up to 2.1 cm thick. The adjacent medial part of gastric fundus is probably mildly involved. No obvious involvement of the distal oesophagus is noted. Nasal gastric tube is noted in-site with its tip at the gastro-oesophageal junction. No obvious perigastric infiltration is seen. No ascites or mesenteric mass is noted. No other bowel thickening is seen in the rest of the abdomen.

Authorized and Reported
on 03-05-2012 @ 20:02 by

MBBS (HK), DMRD (UK), FRCR (UK)
FHKCR, FHKAM (Radiology)

Page 2 of 3

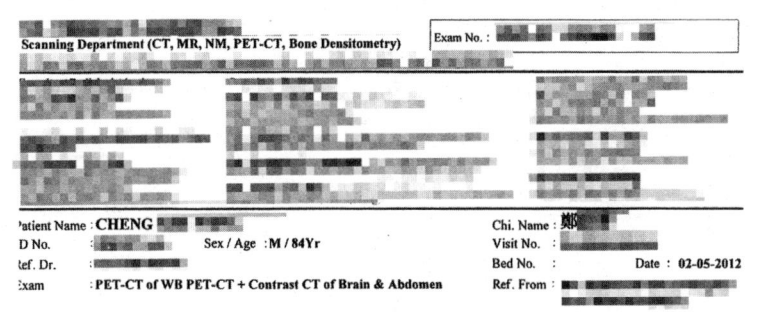

Scanning Department (CT, MR, NM, PET-CT, Bone Densitometry) Exam No. :

Patient Name : CHENG Chi. Name :
D No. : Sex / Age : M / 84Yr Visit No. :
Ref. Dr. : Bed No. : Date : 02-05-2012
Exam : PET-CT of WB PET-CT + Contrast CT of Brain & Abdomen Ref. From :

The liver is normal in size and attenuation. No focal liver lesion is seen. Biliary tree is not dilated. Portal vein is patent. Gallbladder is unremarkable. No calcified gallstone is seen. Gallbladder wall is not thickened.

Spleen is not enlarged. Pancreas is normal in size and attenuation. No pancreatic mass is seen. Pancreatic duct is not dilated. Both kidneys are normal in size and attenuation. A few simple cysts are seen in both kidneys. The largest cyst is seen in the lower pole of right kidney (SE 5 IM 45 film 11). It measures 3.9 x 4.3 cm in transverse diameters. No renal stone or hydronephrosis is seen. Both adrenal glands are not enlarged.

A prominent perigastric lymph node 0.9 cm in size is seen along the lesser curve of stomach (SE 5 IM 24 film 9). It short axis measures less than 1 cm suggestive of reactive lymph although early lymph node metastasis cannot be excluded. No lymphadenopathy is seen in the abdomen. No regional bone erosion is seen. Lung bases are clear.

Comment:

Nodular wall thickening is seen along the upper part of lesser curve of stomach with involvement of the gastro-osephagyeal junction and medial part of gastric fundus consistent with carcinoma of stomach. No obvious perigastric infiltration is seen. A prominent perigastric lymph node is seen along the lesser curve of stomach measuring 0.9 cm. It short axis measures less than 1 cm suggestive of reactive lymph although early lymph node metastasis cannot be excluded. No focal liver lesion is seen. No ascites or mesenteric mass is noted. A few simple cysts are seen in both kidneys. No renal stone or hydronephrosis is seen. Spleen, pancreas and adrenal glands are unremarkable.

Thank you for your referral.

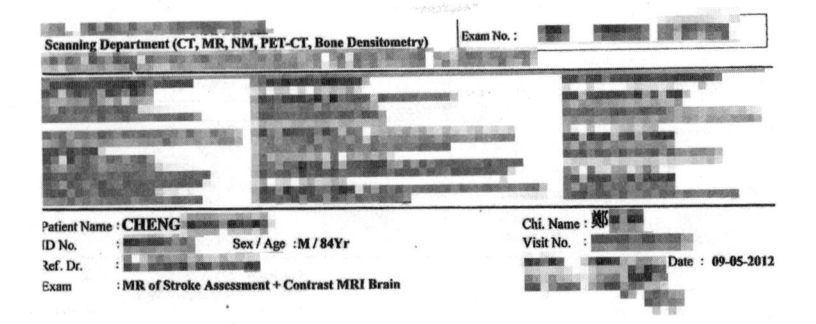

Scanning Department (CT, MR, NM, PET-CT, Bone Densitometry)	Exam No. :

Patient Name : CHENG
ID No. :
Ref. Dr. :
Sex / Age : M / 84Yr
Chi. Name : 鄭
Visit No. :
Date : 09-05-2012
Exam : MR of Stroke Assessment + Contrast MRI Brain

Opinion:

Multiple recent infarcts with diffusion-weighted hyperintense signals are noted at the right corona radiata and subcortical regions of the right fronto-parietal lobes.

The enhancing areas of the right basal ganglia as well as right parietal and frontal cortex are probably also subacute infarcts rather than metastases in view of their lack of mass effect and perifocal oedema. Follow-up study would be most useful for confirmation.

Mild haemorrhagic change is noted at the suspected right parietal infarct. Otherwise, no sizable intracranial haematoma or space-occupying lesion is detected. No definite intracranial metastatic disease is demonstrated.

The MR angiography demonstrates intracranial atherosclerotic changes but no significant steno-occlusive disease is resulted. On the other hand, critical extracranial stenosis is detected at the proximal right internal carotid artery near the carotid bifurcation, measuring more than 80-90% by diameter.

病案 9
命余一至三个月，补正祛邪续新篇

2008年中，79岁的李老太因严重呕吐、呕血，前往医院就诊，经检查患了胃癌，是为第四期即最晚期。她当时吃什么呕什么，甚至饮一小口水也会即时呕吐。因为呕吐中常有黑色血块，导致贫血、全身无力，精神状态极差。

十天后，她又发生严重胸痛，不敢呼吸，气促气短、胸闷，于是再次到医院急诊检查，发现了肿瘤的肺部转移。应诊的马来西亚医院医生对她女儿说，她的年龄太大，病情严重，身体状态又很差，无法接受打击性治疗，预计只剩一至三个月生命了。

仅剩一至三个月生命

李老太一生坎坷，她是马来西亚华侨，六十年前随丈夫从福建移居至马来西亚。她数十年不分日夜，操劳生计，种田养猪，在艰苦的生活中养育了十一个子女。这些年来，子女都已长大，渐渐有了自己的工作和生活，李老太也逐渐感到生活的压力减少。但2008年初，由于老伴去世，她非常伤心，每日哭泣，不想进食，以后又感到下咽困难，呕吐的现象越来越严重。子女们最初以为她伤心过度，慢慢会好的，其后陪伴她到医院检查，才得知是患上了晚期胃癌并有肺淋巴等转移。当子女们获知李老太只剩一至三个月生命时，他们全都伤心悲痛，后悔莫及。

女儿细心刻意瞒病情

她的第九个女儿任职保险业，是此行业的精英。她在生活中对母亲也十分照顾，决心带母亲到香港，寻找新的办法治病救命。于是母女两人乘飞机到香港，再乘车风尘仆仆尽快赶到诊所。李小姐很细心，填写病历时在病历的第一页上，认真写了联络电话、姓名、年龄等。除此之外，她还在下方特意写上一句话："请注意，别让患者知道她的病情，谢谢！"。当时李老太病情很严重，胸痛、腹痛、全身疼痛难忍、气短难续、不时呕吐、并吐黑血、精神很差，不能进食。

李小姐是冒险带母亲乘飞机来就诊的。如果患者知道自己得了晚期胃癌伴有肺转移，精神上会受到很大的打击，加上搭乘飞机的辛苦颠簸，能否承受得了，确实很难说。

李老太只会用难懂的家乡话与女儿沟通，不懂其他语言，也不识字，看诊、问诊也靠女儿翻译。李老太没有一点精神压力，认为只是年岁大了，随女儿找中医调理身体。由于路途遥远，病情严重，医师建议她们先住两天，在此期间一方面服用中药并观察药后反应，一方面加用针灸等方法强化治疗。第二天，李老太的疼痛即有减轻，精神状态有所好转，可以少量进食。于是医师开具了一个月剂量的抗癌中医药，让她们带回家每日服用，以观后效。

治则：扶正祛邪，散结消瘤。

常用中药：人参、仙鹤草、田七、砂仁、厚朴、鸡内金、山楂、青皮、三棱、莪术、桃仁、杏仁、海浮石。

患者年老体弱，用扶助正气的中药是不可少的。同时病邪炽盛，上有双肺转移，中有不能进食、呕吐，下有便血、大便困难，中药需上中下三焦通治，以扶正行滞，散结消瘤。

一个月后，母女俩再次来到香港。与第一次来诊相比，李老太判若两人，身体状态有了明显的改善，就这样，先是一个月来一次，以后两三个月来一次，每次来后治疗一至两天，并带中药回家服用。李老太现已逐渐恢复正常生活，还在家操持家务。

年老体弱难承受化疗

到 2015 年末李老太大脑衰退，在睡眠中平和去世，由当初发现癌病时只剩下一至三个月的生命至此已多活了七年多。不能不承认，抗癌中医药治疗对晚期癌症有非常明确的治疗效果。对于年老体弱、不能承受打击性化疗、手术及放疗的患者更是非常必要的治疗手段。

胃癌是消化道肿瘤中发病率很高的肿瘤，不同地区的发病情况差别很大，例如日本、澳洲、芬兰等国家发病率高，一般认为与环境因素、土壤和饮用水的微量元素含量、工业废物污染、饮食因素、饮食习惯、免疫因素、遗传因素等有关。

对李老太的中医药治疗以补中、降逆、化瘀、软坚为主。当然在长达多年的治疗中，以抗癌中医药治疗为主，并经常根据她的病情做一些调整。

诊疗记录

2009 年 2 月 4 日 CT 报告证实胃癌。

2009 年 2 月 4 日 CT 报告证实有肺转移。

2014 年 2 月，李老太的乖女隔月陪伴来港复诊，战胜癌魔。

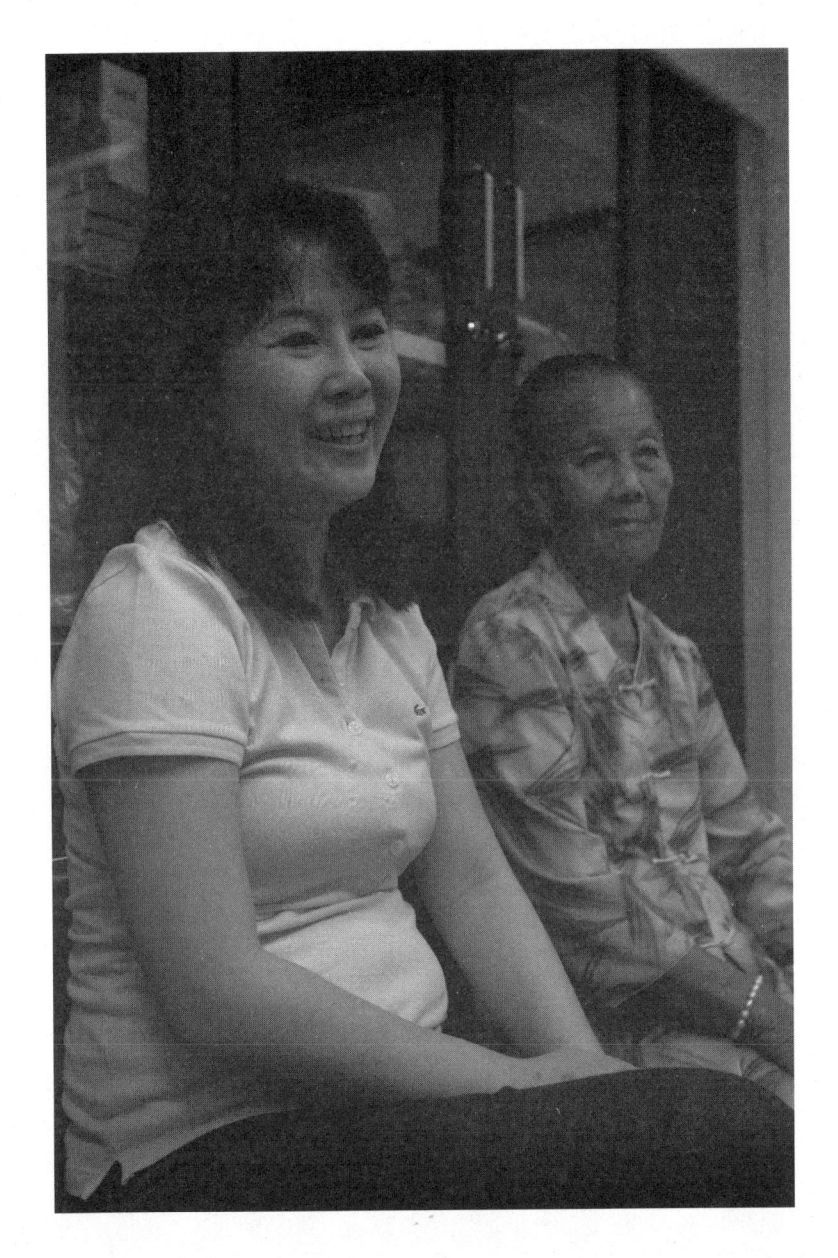

抗癌治验录 下篇

治癌实录 2
中晚期癌症·名家手记

附：患者检查报告

DIAGNOSTIC IMAGING REPORT

NAME	:	TAN
ID NO	:	
SEX	:	FEMALE
AGE	:	80 YEARS
ACCESSION NO	:	
EXAMINATION CATEGORY	:	
ITEM CATEGORY	:	

MRN	:	
ADM/VISIT NO	:	
ADM/VISIT DATE	:	04/02/2009
REPORT TYPE	:	FINAL
EXAMINATION DATE	:	04/02/2009 10:55:11

REPORT : CT ABDOMEN AND PELVIS

Scans at 5 mm intervals were done through the abdomen and pelvis. Oral gastrograffin was given to opacify the bowel.

The liver, pancreas and the spleen are normal. Both kidneys and adrenals are normal in size, shape and position. No enlarged para-aortic or pelvic lymph nodes are seen. No abnormal pelvic mass is noted.

Thickening of gastric wall noted as before.

CONCLUSION

No evidence of metastasis.

SIGNATURE :
NAME :
DESIGNATION : CONSULTANT RADIOLOGIST

Computer generated document.

Print Date/Time : 04/02/2009 15:27:17

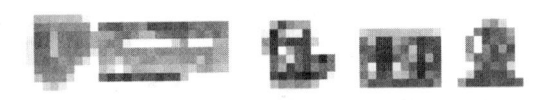

DIAGNOSTIC IMAGING REPORT

NAME	: TAN	**MRN**	:	
		ADM/VISIT NO	:	
ID NO	:	**ADM/VISIT DATE**	:	04/02/2009
SEX	: FEMALE	**REPORT TYPE**	:	FINAL
AGE	: 80 YEARS			
ACCESSION NO	:	**EXAMINATION DATE**	:	04/02/2009 10:55:11
EXAMINATION CATEGORY	:			
ITEM CATEGORY	:			

REPORT : CT CHEST

Post contrast scans at 5 mm thick slices in axial planes were done from the sternal notch down to the epigastrium.

The mass in right middle lobe measures 3 x 1.5cm and is unchanged in size.

There are four small nodules in the right middle lobe measuring < 1cm.

Left lung is clear.

No enlarged lymph node or pleural effusion seen.

CONCLUSION

- No change in the right middle lobe mass measuring 3 x 1.5cm.
- Four small nodules in the right middle lobe are not seen before suggesting new lesions.

SIGNATURE :
NAME :
DESIGNATION : CONSULTANT RADIOLOGIST

Computer generated document.

Print Date/Time : 04/02/2009 15:32:30

病案 10
肝癌劫后获新生

朱女士以前身体状态良好,自认为体质不错,不会得什么重病。但2006年时,她经常感到疲劳、食欲缺乏、体重下降、胁部隐隐作痛。在丈夫的催促下,她去医院做检查,结果令全家都震惊,原来她患了肝癌。

因肿瘤很大,医生建议手术切除。全家经商量决定尽早做手术,于是在2006年10月切除了肝脏。术后宋女士认真接受化疗,但于2007年上半年又复发,未切除的肝脏又长出了肿瘤。经过多处就诊和咨询,朱女士和家人得知病情已非常严重,而且化疗等方法也已无用,资深的医生提出了肝脏移植的办法,朱女士心想,如把长有癌的肝脏全部不要了,换一个健康人的新肝脏,一定就没有癌症了。所以虽然价格昂贵,但大家都认为换了肝就可治愈肝癌,于是全家积极协助医院找寻肝源,做好换肝的各种准备。

换了肝，癌细胞仍然转移

2007年11月，宋女士终于找到了健康的肝源，顺利进行了换肝手术。术后又遵照医生的指示用抗排斥、调整免疫、抗感染等多种治疗，身体恢复得很好，全家人都松了一口气，以为这次可以万事大吉了。

但是好景不长，换肝后仅一年，2008年11月，朱女士又发生了肝癌的肺转移。全家这次深深知道了癌症的可怕，即使患有癌的肝脏已被全部去除，仍然发生了双肺的转移。之后的日子里，朱女士按医生的安排做了化疗、放疗、伽马刀等，将可以使用的手段都用了，肿瘤仍频繁复发、增大，咳嗽、气喘、全身无力等症状越来越重。在这种万般无奈的情况下，朱女士经朋友介绍寻求中医药治疗。当时大家都不以为然，各种现代化的治疗办法都用过了，一些中草药能有多大用处呢？因为没有其他办法，只有先试试了。

症见气喘严重，咳嗽频频连续，没有一分钟停止不咳，纳差、无力、头晕、舌淡红、脉细数。

治则：扶正固本，祛邪抗癌。

常用中药：人参、白术、川大黄、醋鳖甲、炮穿山甲、三棱、莪术、杏仁、青龙衣、重楼、桃仁、红花。消瘤粉、散结丸同时服用。

人参、白术补气补中,三棱、莪术、桃仁、红花行气化瘀,炮穿山甲、重楼、青龙衣软坚祛癌毒,川大黄等排毒通腑。

用肝移植术治疗肝癌,特别是复发的,对于中晚期肝癌效果并不理想。与本例患者同期住院接受同样方法治疗的两个病房的患者在不久的一段时间后都相继离世,就是例证。本例患者接受了换肝手术,术后又有排斥反应及多发性肺转移肿瘤,正虚邪实是很明确的,在十年多的生命修复调治过程中,医师一直密切了解病情,为她详细辨证施治,并根据诊所得到的信息进行扶正治疗,包括养血益肝、补气益肺、固肾补元等,对于双肺的多发转移,采用了散结化痰、化瘀通络、排毒行滞等方法进行治疗。

治疗一段时间后,朱女士精神慢慢好转,咳嗽、气喘也逐渐减少,增强了信心,坚持治疗。以后的几年里,她仍按时去医院定期检查,但没有再复发,医生们也都高兴地对朱女士说,她创造了奇迹。

几位换肝病友先后去世

前些日子，朱女士想起了在同一时期因肝癌而换肝的几位病友，他们在同一时期同一医院住院治疗，相互都很熟悉了，她想联络这几位朋友，但到处打听都得不到他们的消息，后来终于了解到，他们都已于术后半年左右先后离世，因为怕她知道后难过，大家便没有告诉她。

朱女士很明白抗癌中医药治疗效果是真实的，她有信心战胜癌症。从患病至 2016 年 2 月随访已有十年时间了，朱女士每日忙忙碌碌地与朋友一起旅游、参加派对、音乐会，一点也闲不住。之后，朱女士的女儿喜得贵子，她也当上了外婆，朱女士抱着白白胖胖的外孙喜上眉梢，在外孙的出生百日庆贺宴上，还特意拍照片给大家看，以纪念这个难得的时刻。

诊疗记录

2011 年 2 月 11 日 CT 检查报告证实肝癌肝移植手术后，双肺转移病灶与 2010 年对比稳定及无变化。

2012 年 7 月 25 日 CT 检查报告证实肝移植手术后，双肺病灶与以前相比稳定及无变化。

2013 年 6 月，朱女士重获健康新生，并喜获贵孙。

治癌实录 2
中晚期癌症·名家手记

附：患者检查报告

CT 诊断报告

影像号：	住院号：/	科　别：普外科1
姓　名：朱■■ 性　别：女	年　龄：52	病床号：/
检查部位：胸部平扫＋增强		

影像所见：

　　肝移植术后肺转移瘤行放射治疗后：双肺野多发不规则磨玻璃样密度影，其内可见空泡及扩张支气管影，增强后病灶强化；左肺上叶见一微小结节状高密度影，边界清晰，未见强化。两侧局部胸膜增厚粘连改变，肺门形态可，纵隔内未见肿大淋巴结，但可见右侧迷走锁骨下动脉自主动脉弓后部发出。肝移植术后，肝内可见斑点状极高密度影，增强扫描肝内未见异常强化灶，门静脉强化均匀。所见胸廓骨质未见破坏。

影像诊断：

　　左肺上叶微小结节灶治疗后，对比10-11-02老片相仿。
　　双肺多发磨玻璃样病灶，与10-11-02老片相仿，其余病灶与前片相仿。
　　右侧迷走锁骨下动脉。
　　肝移植术后。

报告医师：　　　审核医师：　　　修订医生：

报告时间：2011-02-11 09:29:02

抗癌治验录 下篇

CT 诊断报告

影像号：　　　　　　　　　住院号：　　　　　　科　别：门诊普内科
姓　名：朱**　　性　别：女　　年　龄：53　　病床号：
检查部位：胸部平扫＋增强

影像所见：

　　肝移植术后肺转移瘤行放射治疗后：双肺野多发不规则磨玻璃样密度影，其内可见空泡及扩张支气管影，增强后病灶强化；左肺上叶一微小结节状高密度影，边界清晰，未见强化。两侧局部胸膜增厚粘连改变，肺门形态可，纵隔内未见肿大淋巴结，但可见右侧迷走锁骨下动脉自主动脉弓后部发出在食道后方绕行。肝移植术后，肝内可见斑点状极高密度影，增强扫描肝内未见异常强化灶，门静脉强化均匀。所见胸廓骨质未见破坏。

影像诊断：

　　双肺多发磨玻璃样病灶，对比前片（2012.4.6）相仿，慢性炎症可能。
　　左肺上叶微小结节灶治疗后，对比前片（2012.4.6）相仿。
　　右侧迷走锁骨下动脉。
　　肝移植术后。

报告医师：　　　　审核医师：　　　修订医生：

报告时间：2012-07-25 09:26:20

病案 11
战胜肝癌，喜获麟儿

曾先生于2004年发现患有乙型肝炎，最初不以为意，认为这病只需打针及按医嘱吃药即可康复，但其后又发现有脂肪肝和肝硬化。而这一切亦只是开始。跟一些乙型肝炎患者一样，曾先生于2006年发现肝癌，而且肝癌的指数很高，肿瘤很大。他当时想"这是绝症，没法可医，这次死定了！"，想法非常负面。幸得家人支持，他心情慢慢平复。

曾先生的身体状态逐渐恶化，脸色也开始发黑，不仅肝区疼痛，有时背部也会出现剧烈的疼痛，而且一天当中总要受到几次剧痛的侵袭，痛苦不堪。于是他于2007年1月做了肝癌肿瘤切除手术，心想毒瘤已切除，应该没事了。

曾先生在2007年术后不久就开始进行长时间的化疗。为期一年多的一连串手术及化疗，终于在痛楚的煎熬下完成。刚想松口气，不料于2008年9月，即手术切除肿瘤后一年多，就发现肝脏的肿瘤又长出来了，按医生的意见需要再切除肿瘤及做化疗。

有位当医生的朋友告诉曾先生，再次切除或再化疗后，肿瘤仍有机会复发。这对曾先生无疑是个非常大的打击，也令他的意志逐渐消沉。虽然家人对他说："你曾经战胜过病魔，这次也一定可以的！"但才短短一年就复发，曾先生不得不重新萌生了无法战胜癌症的想法。在住院期间，曾先生看见身边的癌症病友一个个先他而去感到相当畏惧，一切似乎无能为力。

肝炎指数转为正常

幸好家人一直没有放弃，深信存在痊愈的机会，曾先生也没有再次切除肿瘤，而是经朋友介绍，选择了生命修复抗癌中医药治疗。

就诊见，右胁刺痛，精神疲惫，消瘦，腹胀嗳气，恶心、纳差、呕吐、下肢水肿，脉弦细，舌暗苔腻。

治则：化瘀软坚，健脾利湿。

常用中药：柴胡、鳖甲、丹参、莪术、三棱、党参、茯苓、土鳖虫、猪苓。散结丸同时服用。

肝癌的用药，应根据患者正气、邪毒两方面各自的盛衰来决定，体质较强，正气未衰，邪毒亢盛之时，可攻伐，以行气、化瘀、攻坚为主；正气已衰，体质虚弱，则先培补正气，以健脾、补肾、养肝为主。或攻补兼施、补多攻少、攻多补少，总以具体辨证分析，来进行精准的治疗。

治疗至今，曾先生的病情已趋稳定，肿瘤没有复发，乙型肝炎的指数也转为正常。

2011年初，曾先生感到身体状态良好，他已四十多岁，但一直膝下无子，除了抗癌外，也道出了想要个孩子的想法。于是他除了接受抗癌中医药治疗外，也同时做身体调理，扶正祛邪、培补肾精。曾先生通过中医药调理，身体有了全方位好转，并于2012年5月喜获麟儿。如今他的儿子五岁多了，本人患癌至今也有十一年了，他深有感触地说，是抗癌中医药治疗给了他新的生活和生命。

诊疗记录

2007年1月20日肝肿瘤切除后病理报告，证实为肝细胞癌。

2009年12月16日MRI检查报告，肝有新生结节（同时AFP升高）考虑肿瘤复发。

2011年7月8日，乙型肝炎病毒DNA为阳性。

2012年2月3日，乙型肝炎病毒DNA为阴性。

2012年11月23日MRI，Scan检查报告显示，肝癌没有复发和转移。

2013年4月，曾先生的肝癌再无复发，更喜获麟儿。

抗癌治验录 下篇

附：患者检查报告

PATIENT'S NAME		DATE RECEIVED	PATHOLOGY NO.	COPY:
曾 CHANG		20/01/2007		'DR. HOSP OTHERS
I.D. NO.	SEX M	AGE 39 Y	PREVIOUS PATH. NO.	
HOSPITAL	HOSPITAL NO.	CLASS		

UNDER CARE OF DR.	
DOCTOR'S ADDRESS	
CLINICAL PROCEDURE	Excision right lobe liver tumour.
CLINICAL SUMMARY	Segment 5 and segment 8 resection. Specimens segment 5, segment 8, gall bladder.
FROZEN SECTION DIAGNOSIS (if any)	---
PATHOLOGICAL DIAGNOSIS	(1) Right lobe liver (segmentectomy) - Moderately differentiated hepatocellular carcinoma, completely excised. (2) Gall bladder (cholecystectomy) - Benign.

REPORT

Macroscopic examination:

(1) "Segment 5 + 8 of liver" - Two pieces of liver tissue altogether 280 grams in weight, 12 x 9 x 5 cm., 7 x 5.5 x 4.7 cm. The larger piece, partly cut-open before receipt, showed a well-defined firm tan-coloured nodular tumour 3 x 1.8 x 1.8 cm. which was 1.1 cm. from the resection margin. The capsular surface of the liver was grossly intact. The smaller piece of liver tissue showed no definite macroscopic lesions on sectioning.

(2) "Gall bladder" - A green-brown smooth-surfaced gall bladder 7.5 cm. long, 3 cm. in diameter. On sectioning the mucosa was green-brown and intact and the wall measured 0.2 to 0.3 cm. thick. No stones were received.

Microscopic examination:

(1) Sections of the tumour show a moderately differentiated hepatocellular carcinoma with trabecular and focal pseudoglandular morphology. The tumour is multinodular, but no definite microsatellite foci are seen in adjacent hepatic parenchyma. Some dilated peritumoural lymphatics show tumour emboli without definite mural invasion. The capsular surface and resection margins are clear. Adjacent liver parenchyma shows an established cirrhosis, with minimal interface hepatitis, and extensive macrovesicular steatosis. The smaller piece of liver tissue shows no evidence of malignancy.

(2) Gall bladder shows no significant pathological abnormalities.

Date Reported: 22/01/2007   Signed:

治癌实录 2

中晚期癌症・名家手记

Name: CHANG,
Sex/Age/DOB: M/42/
Ref.Dr.:
Exam ID.:

ID No.:
Room/Bed:
Hospital No.:
Date of Exam: 16 Dec, 2009

MRI SCAN OF ABDOMEN WITH AND WITHOUT CONTRAST

Clinical data: Ca liver resected.

Technique:
Pre-contrast:
Axial T1, T2, fat-sat T2, fat-sat T1
Coronal T2 weighted
Axial long fat-sat T2, in & out-of-phase

Post-contrast (Gadolinium):
Dynamic Axial fat saturation T1 weighted
Coronal fat saturation T1 weighted

Findings:
Comparison is made with previous MRI dated 26 May 2009.

Evidence of previous right hepatectomy is noted. Left lobe liver remnant is hypertrophied.

There is a small T1 slightly hyperintense and T2 isointense nodule in anterior aspect of left lateral segment. It shows signal loss in the opposed-phase image, suggestive of presence of intralesional fat. After contrast injection, no significant arterial enhancement is seen. It is hypoenhancing in the portovenous and delayed phase (series 16 image 40 and series 19 image 17). It is not seen in previous MRI.

No other focal mass lesion in the liver is demonstrated. Portal veins, hepatic veins and IVC are patent.

Bile ducts are not dilated. Spleen is not enlarged. No focal lesion in spleen is seen.

Both adrenal glands are normal. Left kidney is displaced inferiorly due to hypertrophied left lobe of liver. Both kidneys are otherwise normal.

No enlarged retroperitoneal lymphadenopathy is seen. No ascites is present.

Impression:
1. Status post right hepatectomy. Hypertrophied left lobe liver remnant.
2. Tiny fat containing nodule without significant arterial enhancement in anterior aspect of left lateral segment. It is not seen in previous MRI dated 26 May 2009. DDx include focal fat deposit, regenerative nodule or recurrent hepatocellular carcinoma. Suggest correlation with AFP and close follow-up MRI for progress.

Department of Diagnostic & Interventional Radiology
MBChB FRCR FHKCR FHKAM (Radiology)

抗癌治验录 下篇

Name	Chang			
Age/Gender	40Y/M	D.O.B.		
File No		I.D. No		
Drawn	July 8, 2011 12:33 PM			
Received	July 8, 2011 12:32 PM			
Reported	July 11, 2011 2:53 PM			
Lab No				
Remarks				
Specimen	All samples are blood, unless otherwise indicated.			

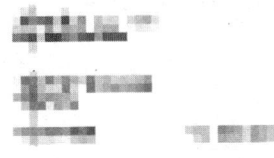

Hepatitis B Virus DNA (by PCR) 乙型肝炎病毒DNA   8.4 IU/mL 4.89×10^1 copies/mL

Interpretation of results :

Not detected	HBV DNA not detected. However, an "undetected" HBV DNA test result does not exclude the presence of past or resolved HBV infection.
< 20 IU/mL	HBV DNA is detected but is < 20 IU/mL. The HBV DNA level present is below the quantifiable lower limit of this assay.
20 - 1.7×10^8 IU/mL	HBV DNA detected. Calculated results are within the linear range of the test.
> 1.7×10^8 IU/mL	HBV DNA is detected but is >1.70×10^8 IU/mL. The level of HBV DNA present is above the quantifiable upper limit of this assay.

Reference notes:
The assay used is the COBAS AmpliPrep / TaqMan (FDA-approved) in-vitro assay. Due to its high sensitivity, this assay is useful for detecting some cases of early acute HBV infection (before the appearance of HBsAg), to distinguish replicative from nonreplicative chronic HBV infection, and to monitor patient's response to anti-HBV therapy.

It is not unusual for HBeAg '+' patients to have millions of HBV DNA. Therefore results are reported in "log" format. For monitoring, a significant change is generally > 2 log change. This compensates for the inherent variability in PCR assays, as well as physiologic variation and concurrent illnesses in the HBV-infected patients. Significant levels of virus prior to treatment depend on HBeAg +/- and ALT levels and other factors.[1]

Ref:
1. Keeffe, E.B., Dieterich, D.T., Han, S.H.B., Jacobson, I.M., Martin, P., Schiff, E.R., Tobias, H., A Treatment Algorithm for the Management of Chronic Hepatitis B Virus Infection in the United States:2006 Update, Clinical Gastroenterology and Hepatology (2008), doi: 10.1016/j.cgh.2008.08.021.
2. Roche Molecular Systems Inc., Cobas AmpliPrep / TaqMan HBV System Package Insert : Ref 05382814001-01 (11/2008)

Approved signatory :

Printed : Jul 11, 2011 15:08:08

治癌实录 2
中晚期癌症·名家手记

Name	Chang		
Age/Gender	44Y/M	D.O.B.	
File No		I.D. No	
Drawn	February 3, 2012 4:24 PM		
Received	February 3, 2012 4:23 PM		
Reported	February 6, 2012 3:15 PM		
Lab No			
Remarks			
Specimen	All samples are blood, unless otherwise indicated.		

Hepatitis B Virus DNA (by PCR) 乙型肝炎病毒DNA   Not detected

Interpretation of results :

Not detected	HBV DNA not detected. However, an "undetected" HBV DNA test result does not exclude the presence of past or resolved HBV infection.
< 20 IU/mL	HBV DNA is detected but is < 20 IU/mL. The HBV DNA level present is below the quantifiable lower limit of this assay.
20 - 1.7 x 10^8 IU/mL	HBV DNA detected. Calculated results are within the linear range of the test.
> 1.7 x 10^8 IU/mL	HBV DNA is detected but is >1.70 x 10^8 IU/mL. The level of HBV DNA present is above the quantifiable upper limit of this assay.

Reference notes:
The assay used is the COBAS AmpliPrep / TaqMan (FDA-approved) in-vitro assay. Due to its high sensitivity, this assay is useful for detecting some cases of early acute HBV infection (before the appearance of HBsAg), to distinguish replicative from nonreplicative chronic HBV infection, and to monitor patient's response to anti-HBV therapy.

It is not unusual for HBeAg '+' patients to have millions of HBV DNA. Therefore results are reported in "log" format. For monitoring, a significant change is generally > 2 log change. This compensates for the inherent variability in PCR assays, as well as physiologic variation and concurrent illnesses in the HBV-infected patients. Significant levels of virus prior to treatment depend on HBeAg +/- and ALT levels and other factors.[1]

Ref:
1. Keeffe, E.B., Dieterich, D.T., Han, S.H.B., Jacobson, I.M., Martin, P., Schiff, E.R., Tobias, H., A Treatment Algorithm for the Management of Chronic Hepatitis B Virus Infection in the United States:2008 Update, Clinical Gastroenterology and Hepatology (2008), doi: 10.1016/j.cgh.2008.08.021.
2. Roche Molecular Systems Inc., Cobas AmpliPrep / TaqMan HBV System Package Insert : Ref 05302814001-01 (11/2008)

Approved signatory :

Printed : Feb 6, 2012

診斷及介入放射部
Department of Diagnostic & Interventional Radiology

Name: CHANG.
Sex / DOB: M /
Referrer:
Exam ID(s):

ID:
Ward / Dept: Clinicians
Hosp No.:
Date of Exam: 23-NOV-2012

MRI SCAN OF ABDOMEN WITH AND WITHOUT CONTRAST

Clinical data:
Ca liver resected. Hepatitis B.

Technique:

Pre-contrast:
Axial T1, T2, T2 fat-sat, T1 fat-saturation
Coronal T2 weighted

Post-contrast (Gadolinium):
Axial T1 fat saturation
Coronal T1 fat saturation

Findings:
Comparison is made with previous examination performed in February 2012. The right lobe of liver is absent. Hypertrophy of liver remnant is noted. It shows homogeneous signal intensity. No abnormal mass is present. No abnormal arterial enhancing lesion to suggest hepatoma is present.
The biliary ducts are not dilated. Gallbladder is absent.
Portal vein is patent. No thrombosis is present.
The kidneys are normal in size and outline. No abnormal mass is present. No hydronephrosis is noted.
The pancreas is normal in appearance. No pancreatic lesion is present. Pancreatic duct is not dilated.
Spleen is not enlarged.
Bowel structures have normal pattern. No abnormal bowel lesion is present. No obvious bowel mass is noted.
No significant adenopathy is present. No mesenteric adenopathy is noted.
No free peritoneal fluid is present.
Limited scan of both lung bases reveals no abnormal pulmonary masses.

Impression:
1. Hepatocellular carcinoma, status post right hepatectomy. No MR evidence of recurrence.
2. No intra-abdominal metastatic lesion is noted.

MBBS DMRD FRCR FHKCR FHKAM(Radiology)

Typed By :

Approved Date-Time:
23-NOV-2012 05:16 PM

Received at _____ Time _____ Ready by Dr. _____ Signature _____ Date _____ Time _____
   dd/mm/yy   dd/mm/yy

病案 12
消瘤扶正，正常生活

　　胰腺癌是消化系统常见高度恶性肿瘤，由于肿瘤生长速度和发展都极快，目前尚缺乏有效的治疗，一般认为其发生率与死亡率几乎相同，有"癌中之王"之称。西医通常会明确地告知家人此病的严重性，说明可做手术，但预后不好，生存时间不长。邓女士于 2010 年 3 月做了胰腺癌的切除手术。正如所料，术后的病理检查报告显示，病情严重，很不乐观。胰头部的癌症已包裹并侵入门静脉，肿瘤已侵入十二指肠固有肌层和周围神经。更没想到的是，一般手术切除肿瘤时会尽量多切除一些周围的正常组织，以免肿瘤切不干净，但是邓女士的检查报告显示，切除的癌瘤非常接近周围的组织，距离切缘仅有 0.01 厘米，就是说几乎没有切下周围的正常组织。这种情况下，肿瘤复发和转移的概率是极大的，所以手术后医院要求她尽快进行化疗和放疗。

　　家人经过一番了解和查询，得知胰腺癌的化疗和放疗并无明确效果，于是下决心不做化疗和放疗了。邓女士在家人陪同下前来诊所进行生命修复中心抗癌治疗。

就诊时症见精神极差、消瘦、倦怠乏力、面白无华、脘腹胀痛、嗳气呕吐、不能进食、大便少，舌淡红，脉沉细数。

治则：补血益气，消肿散结。

常用中药：人参、当归、白芍、赤芍、茯苓、生薏苡仁、猫爪草、鸡内金、八月札、龙葵、炒麦芽。消瘤2号同时服用。

经治疗后，邓女士的病情明显好转，腹痛也逐渐缓解，进食增多，体重渐增，慢慢恢复了正常生活。

多年来，每年去复查都未见有转移复发，邓女士自诊断患有胰腺癌至今已有八年了，她生活愉快，与儿孙一起住，尽享天伦之乐。

治癌实录 2
中晚期癌症·名家手记

附：患者检查报告

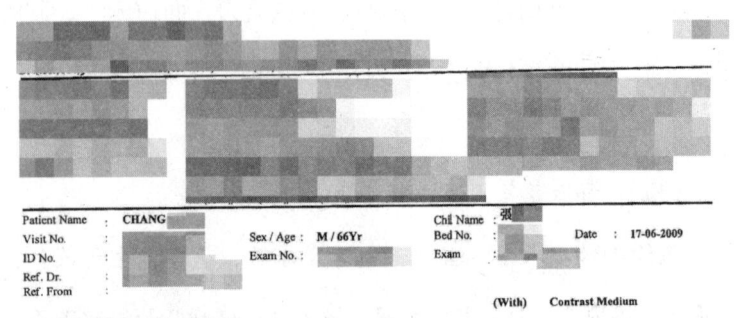

Patient Name :	CHANG		Chi Name :		
Visit No. :		Sex / Age : M / 66Yr	Bed No. :	Date :	17-06-2009
ID No. :		Exam No. :	Exam		
Ref. Dr. :					
Ref. From :			(With)	Contrast Medium	

Clinical Information / History:

Abdominal shadow in liver. Epigastric pain.
To screen for tumour in the liver, gallbladder and pancreas

Radiological Report:

Imaging Technique:

Pre-contrast 10 mm axial helical scans.
Post-contrast 5 mm axial helical scans at arterial, portovenous and delayed phases.
Multiplanar reformation over regions of interest.

Imaging Findings:

A large necrotic liver mass is found at the anterior segments (segments 7 and 8) of the right hepatic lobe, bulging into the adjacent segment 4b. The liver mass which measures 111 mm x 110 mm in transaxial diameters and 98 mm in height demonstrates prominent contrast enhancement during the arterial phase with rapid contrast washout. It is most likely to be hepatocellular carcinoma but histological study is needed for confirmation.

The right portovenous branches appear obliterated by the large right hepatic tumour. The main portal vein as well as the left portal branch are still patent. The biliary tree is not dilated. A small transient arterial enhancing liver focus is found at subcapsular region of segment 2, measuring 4 mm in diameter. It might represent arterioportal shunt rather than HCC focus. Follow-up study would be most useful for confirmation. The tiny non-enhancing cystic area at the lateral segment is likely to be a simple liver cyst. The liver has coarsened parenchymal enhancement suspicious of liver cirrhosis. No portal hypertension is yet noted. The spleen is not enlarged. No varices or ascites is seen. No sizable lymphadenopathy is noted at the porta hepatis and paraaortic region.

NO. OF FILMS	14	14" x 17"		(DDMM) (HHMM)	REPORT & FILMS SENT OUT :	
NO. OF COLOR PRINT		NO. OF CDR 1	'WET' FILMS: SENT RETURNED		17-06-2009	PM OK
Remark :						

Report No. :

Authorized and Reported
on 17-06-2009 @ 18:35 by

CT, MR, Neuro & Interventional, MBBS (HK), DMRD (UK)
FRCR (UK), FHKCR, FHKAM (Radiology)

on 17-06-2009 @ 18:35:52   Page 1 of 2   Version No. 2

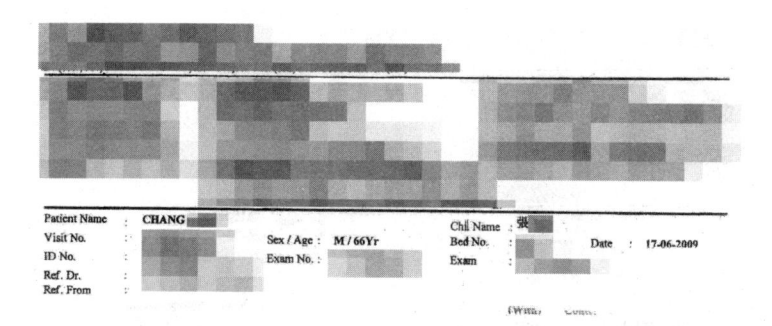

Patient Name	:	CHANG			Chi. Name	:	張		
Visit No.	:		Sex / Age	: M / 66Yr	Bed No.	:		Date	: 17-06-2009
ID No.	:		Exam No.	:	Exam	:			
Ref. Dr.	:								
Ref. From	:								

The gallbladder is normal and no calcified stone is noted. The pancreas shows no sign of inflammation or tumour. The pancreatic duct is not dilated. The adrenal glands are normal in outlines. No abnormal gastric or bowel wall thickening is noted. Both kidneys are small in size with a number of simple renal cortical cysts, suggestive of chronic parenchymal disease. No solid renal mass lesion is present. No hydronephrosis is seen. No calcified renal stone is noted.

No active pulmonary lesion or pleural effusion is noted at the lung bases as included in present study. No regional bony abnormality is noted.

OPINION:

A large necrotic hypervascular tumour is found at the anterior segments of right hepatic lobe, pulsing into the adjacent segment 4b. The imaging features are highly suggestive of hepatocellular carcinoma. The small transient arterial enhancing focus at segment 2 might be arterioportal shunt rather than HCC focus.

The right portovenous branches are obliterated but the main portal vein is still patent. Mild liver cirrhosis is suggested. No portal hypertension is yet evident. No extrahepatic metastatic disease is detected at the upper abdomen. No sizable upper lymphadenopathy or ascites is present. Both kidneys are small with cortical cysts, suggestive of chronic parenchymal disease.

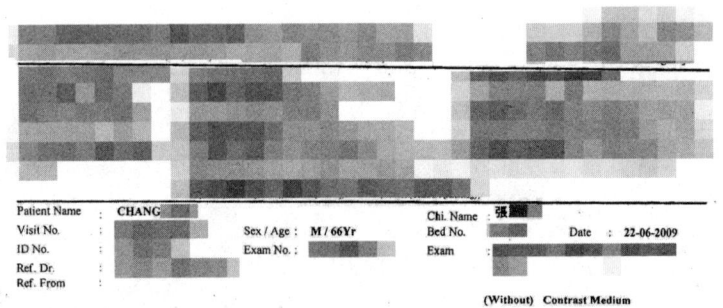

Patient Name	: CHANG			Chi. Name	: 張		
Visit No.	:	Sex / Age :	M / 66Yr	Bed No.	:	Date :	22-06-2009
ID No.	:	Exam No. :		Exam	:		
Ref. Dr.	:						
Ref. From	:			(Without)	Contrast Medium		

Clinical Information / History:

Large right HCC and small left lobe. Plan for SIRTEX.

Radiological Report:

Diagnostic hepatic angiogram is performed by ▓▓▓. The common hepatic artery was identified with X-ray technique. Then, about 3.8 mCi Tc-99m MAA was injected to the common hepatic artery. After hemostasis, the patient was transferred to the scanning department for whole body planar images and SPECT images of the upper abdomen.

FINDINGS

Planar images of the whole body demonstrate no significant uptake in both lungs. There is no significant shunting to the GI tract. Mild physiological tracer activity is noted in the salivary glands, stomach, thyroid, kidneys and bladder, likely due to free technetium.

Planar and SPECT images of the liver demonstrate concentration of MAA in the right hepatic tumour and mild activity in the normal-looking liver tissue. Distribution of blood flow is mildly heterogeneous in the tumour. The tumour to normal liver uptake ratio is about 4:1.

IMPRESSION

There is no significant shunting to the lungs and GI tract. The right hepatic tumour is hypervascular. The tumour to normal liver uptake ratio is about 4:1.

Thank you for your referral.

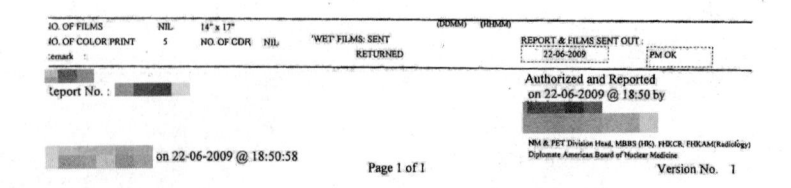

抗癌治验录 下篇

Doctor's Copy

X-Ray & Ultrasound Department

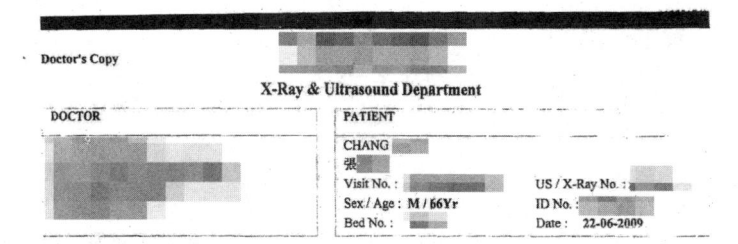

DOCTOR

PATIENT
CHANG
张
Visit No. :
Sex / Age : M / 66Yr
Bed No. :
US / X-Ray No. :
ID No. :
Date : 22-06-2009

Clinical Information / History :

Hepatocellular carcinoma. Large HCC, plain for Sirtex.

X-Ray / Ultrasound Report :

HEPATIC ANGIOGRAM

Right femoral approach with insertion of 5Fr. vascular sheath into the right femoral artery. 4Fr. Cobra I catheter is used for diagnostic angiograms. 5Fr. Yashiro catheter is used for cannulation of the common hepatic artery. Micro-catheter (renegade) is used for selected cannulation and embolization of the gastro-duodenal artery (GDA) and right gastric artery (RGA) and infusion of MAA particle at the distal proper hepatic artery.

On the SMA arterio-portogram and coeliac angiogram, the portal system is patent. On the coeliac angiogram, a sizable vascular mass is seen in inferior right lobe of liver with likely involvement of the medial left lobe. No arterio-portal shunt or arterio-venous shunt is noted. Original of the GAD and RGA are closed to the distal bifurcation of the proper hepatic artery. Both the GDA and RGA are embolized with micro-colis (5 micro-coils for GAD and 3 micro-coils for RGA). Satisfactory result is noted (film 4). The micro-catheter is position at the distal proper hepatic artery just proximal to its bifurcation into the right hepatic artery and left hepatic artery and this is followed by infusion of MAA particles. No immediate complication is noted.

COMMENT:

An hyper-vascular mass is seen in inferior right lobe of liver with likely involvement of the medial left lobe. The portal vein is patent. Origins of the GDA and RGA are quite close to the distal bifurcation of the proper hepatic artery and they are embolized with micro-coils with satisfactory result. MAA particles infused through micro-catheter which is positioned at the distal proper hepatic artery just proximal to its bifurcation. Uneventful procedure.

Report No. :

on 23-06-2009 @ 08:45:24

Authorized and Reported
on 23-06-2009 @ 08:45 by

M.B.B.S.(H.K.),D.M.R.D.(U.K.),F.R.C.R.(U.K.)

Page 1 of 1

Version No.

病案 13

抗乳癌加保胎，母子平安

林小姐留学澳洲，1999年毕业后留在当地工作和生活，她和丈夫一直想要孩子，但多年来一直未能如愿。到2006年，林小姐三十岁时终于有喜了。夫妻俩很高兴，商量为小宝宝准备衣物、营养品。然而怀孕后不久，林小姐便感到两侧乳房胀痛并有肿胀物，她以为是妊娠的正常反应，但为慎重起见，还是去了医院做检查，结果发现两边乳房都各有一个肿块。医生称是良性的乳腺纤维瘤，要她尽早进行手术切除，以免影响以后哺乳。

用药一周后腹痛减少

据医生所讲，因为是良性肿瘤，手术切口很小，仅将肿瘤取出即可，不需要做大面积切除，对乳腺组织也不会有损伤和影响。于是林小姐做了双侧乳腺的小手术将肿瘤取出，以为从此万事大吉。没想到几天后医生又来电话，要她尽快再次做手术，原来切除的两个肿瘤经过检验，右侧为纤维瘤，而左侧为乳腺癌，同时已发生淋巴转移，要尽快较大面积地切除受到恶性肿瘤影响的周围组织，并将腋下等转移的淋巴组织一并切除。

澳洲的医生说化验结果显示肿瘤恶性程度很高，要求林小姐先做流产再进行手术和化疗。林小姐听后如晴天霹雳，她怎么也不敢相信自己得了癌症，更不敢相信要做流产除掉胎儿。她反复恳求医生，希望能够保住胎儿，但是医生的回答很坚决，一定要流产，这是唯一的选择，否则连大人也保不住。林小姐走投无路，联系香港的父母和亲朋，请他们帮助打听有无其他办法。很快得到香港的回复，提及中医药治癌的事情。林小姐当即决定马上来香港，只要有一丝希望，她都要去尝试。

林小姐于2006年5月初来到香港求诊，当时怀孕十九周，由于长途奔波加上心情紧张、悲伤劳累，导致腹痛，胎动不安，有流产的症状。舌淡，脉弦细。抗癌中医药治疗与西药大不相同，可尽量在医治肿瘤的同时，避免流产。

治则：固肾安胎，解郁疏肝，散结攻毒。

常用中药：菟丝子、桑寄生、阿胶、川续断、佛手、白芍、蜂房、海藻、昆布、青龙衣、贝母。消瘤丸同时服用。

菟丝子、桑寄生、川续断益肝肾，固冲任，有安胎功效，又可疏通经络；佛手、白芍解郁疏肝柔肝；海藻、昆布、青龙衣、贝母等散结抗癌。

治则：软坚散结，祛湿解毒。

常用中药：土茯苓、蛇蜕、蝉蜕、僵蚕、牡蛎、鳖甲、急性子、藤梨根等。

蛇蜕、蝉衣走表行皮解毒，土茯苓除湿泄热，通透经络，搜剔湿热之蕴毒；藤梨根利湿解毒，软坚散结，消积抗癌。

治疗一周后，林小姐的腹痛减少，以后继续治疗，抗癌、保胎同时进行，患者精神好转，心情也逐渐变开朗。至2006年9月下旬，喜得麟儿。

患者生产以后，乳腺会分泌大量乳汁，这对乳腺癌患者来说是非常严峻的考验，治疗稍有不妥，病情就会急剧加重并加快转移。但借助医师丰富的治疗经验和正确的抗癌中医药治疗方法，患者终于闯过了这道难关，母子平安。

现在十一年过去了，林小姐仍坚持接受抗癌中医药治疗，她的儿子也有十一岁了，母子生活愉快。林小姐也已在香港工作多年，她很注重儿子的成长，一有时间就带他去学习不同课程、游玩。林小姐从未做过化疗和放疗，甚至澳洲医生严格要求的，需要大面积切除恶性肿瘤和腋部转移淋巴结及周围组织，也完全没有做。靠着抗癌中医药治疗，她终于战胜了癌症。

林小姐，30岁，2006年4月19日澳洲医生写信证实林小姐怀孕17周，并患乳腺癌，淋巴转移，要尽快做化疗及放射治疗。

2006年11月7日（分娩后2个月）PET-CT扫描报告证实患者拒绝化疗。左乳腺和腋下无肿瘤复发，右侧乳腺、腋下、淋巴及头、颈、胸、腹、骨盆、骨骼等部位均没有肿瘤转移和复发。

诊疗记录

2008年4月12日检查报告没有肿瘤复发。

2016年5月，仍看着儿子健康成长。

治癌实录 2
中晚期癌症・名家手记

附：患者检查报告

Institute of Oncology

Department of Medical Oncology

　　　　　　　　　　　　　　　　　　　Hospital
　　　　　　　　　　　　　　　　　　　2031
　　　　　　　　　　　　　　　Tel:
　　　　　　　　　　　　　　　Fax:

MF : mam

19 April 2006

Dr ████████
66████████
████████ NSW 2031

RE: ████████   DOB: ██/██/75

Many thanks for asking me to see Mrs Lam who is 30 years old, 17 weeks pregnant and has recently been diagnosed with an early breast cancer.

She presented with a left breast lump that she thought had been present for over a year but has recently increased in size. On ultrasound she was noted to have an irregular lobulated solid lesion at the 2 o'clock position and the fine needle biopsy was suspicious.

She had a wide local excision and axillary node dissection and the pathology report confirmed a 17mm Grade 2 infiltrating ductal cancer that was oestrogen receptor positive, progesterone receptor positive, Her-2 negative. 2 of 25 axillary nodes were involved.

Mrs Lam has made an uneventful postoperative recovery and was well and asymptomatic when I spoke with her.

She plans to leave Sydney over the weekend and return to Hong Kong where all her family are and I understand has made an appointment to see the breast unit at Queen Mary Hospital in Hong Kong. She will need to have an ultrasound of her liver and chest x-ray with shielding as basic staging and will have these in Hong Kong.

I have had a long talk with her about the approach that we would take to management of early breast cancer in pregnancy. In general, we would manage her as we would a non-pregnant woman with the exception of imaging and avoiding radiation during pregnancy. Adjuvant chemotherapy appears safe during the 2nd and 3rd trimesters and should be considered where clinically indicated.

The general experience of chemotherapy during pregnancy is that foetal malformations are very uncommon in women treated in the 2nd and 3rd trimester. The possible consequences of chemotherapy during pregnancy include intrauterine growth retardation and low birth weight, but as far as one

A FACILITY OF THE SOUTH EASTERN SYDNEY AREA HEALTH SERVICE

抗癌治验录 下篇

can tell late effects appear to be very uncommon. The largest series of follow up was reported from Mexico where 84 women who had chemotherapy during pregnancy had their children followed for a medium of 18 years. There were no cancers or second malignancies in any child. The learning and educational performance was normal and there were no psychological sequelae and no cardiac dysfunction in the children of women who received chemotherapy during pregnancy which is very reassuring. I've explained to Mrs Lam that there is a very useful website on the hospital for sick children in Toronto http://www.motherrisk.org/ that provides a lot of evidence regarding chemotherapy during pregnancy and also there is an international registry of cancer in pregnancy.

I explained that it has been our policy to use a very similar protocol that reported by the Md Anderson Cancer Centre using adjuvant 5-Fluorouracil, Adriamycin and Cyclophosphamide every 3 weeks. We monitor the patients very carefully during pregnancy with regular foetal ultrasounds and work in close conjunction with the Obstetrician and Neonatologist. We tend to deliver the baby at around 33 weeks or so but base this on advice from the Neonatologist and Obstetrician. We plan delivery so it is at least 3 weeks after chemotherapy to avoid delivery when the patients' blood count may be low and we always check the full blood count of the baby after delivery as well.

I have tried to reassure her the best I can and I hope that she will be able to have adjuvant treatment in Hong Kong. I have also explained to her that given the fact that the tumour was strongly oestrogen receptor positive and progesterone receptor positive that she will require hormonal therapy following delivery and this may include an LHRH agonist as well as Tamoxifen. She of course will also need radiotherapy to the breast following chemotherapy.

Professor of Medicine
Conjoint, University of

▮▮▮▮▮ Hospital

Scanning Department
(CT, MR, NM, PET Scan, Bone Densitometry)

PET-CT ▮▮▮▮
EXAM. DATE 7 Nov, 2006

REPORT FOR MRI/CT/NM/PET SCANNING EXAMINATION

NAME Lam ▮▮ ▮▮
ID No. K47▮▮ ▮ **AGE** 30 **SEX** F
EXAM. PET-CT of
FDG - Whole Body Trunk
HOSPITAL ▮▮▮▮▮▮▮▮

CLINICAL HISTORY:

T1N1 Ca breast with left lumpectomy and axillary dissection done in Apr 2006. Refused adjuvant chemo RT. PET-CT for progress.

Blood glucose level is 5.0 mmol/l.

RADIOLOGICAL REPORT:

RADIOPHARMACEUTICAL:

10.6 mCi F-18 deoxyglucose.

FINDINGS:

Whole body trunk PET scan was performed from the base of skull to the upper thighs. Serial tomographic images of the whole body trunk were presented in transaxial, coronal and sagittal projections. Plain CT of whole body trunk was performed for image fusion with PET scan.

No recurrent tumour is identified in the left breast and left axilla. The right breast, right axilla and internal mammary chain are not involved. No abnormal uptake is present in the mediastinum. No hypermetabolic nodule is present in the lungs. The head and neck and supraclavicular fossae are clear.

The liver shows uniform physiological activity. The spleen, adrenals, pancreas and other abdominal and pelvis visceral organs are unremarkable. Incidentally, mild focal uptake is present at the right iliac area, with SUV max. = 3.39. This is probably a reactive lymph node. Follow up assessment is recommended.

No focal lesion is present in the axial skeleton.

(The plain CT images are performed for anatomical correlation and localization of lesion seen on PET. This is not a complete diagnostic contrast CT study).

(SUV = Standardized Glucose Uptake Value.)

IMPRESSION :

FDG PET-CT scan demonstrates no evidence of recurrent tumour in the left breast and left axillae. The right breast, right axilla and internal mammary chain are unremarkable. No recurrent tumour is present in the head and neck, thorax, abdomen, pelvis and axial bony skeleton.

Thank you for your referral.

(This examination does not include the brain.)

SIGNED
DR. ▮▮▮▮▮▮▮

抗癌治验录 下篇

███ Hospital ███ 醫院
MEDICAL IMAGING DEPARTMENT

Patient's Name : LAM ███
Unit Record No : ███

Sex : Female
Age : ███
Examination Date : 12/04/2008
Examination No : ███
Ward / Class : ███

EXAMINATION / PROCEDURE REPORT

Examination : MM/Mammogram - Bilateral

BILATERAL MAMMOGRAM

The parenchymal density of both breasts is dense.
Architectural distortion in the upper outer quadrant of the left breast related to pr
operation is detected.
No focal nodule, suspicious microcalcification, skin thickening or nipple retraction co
detected on both sides.
The axillary regions are unremarkable.

IMPRESSION

Architectural distortion in the upper outer quadrant of the left breast related to pre
operation.
No mammographic evidence of malignancy.
Comparing with the previous study on 10.11.06, no significant interval change is det
Follow up mammogram and ultrasound is recommended.

Statistical Information
6-10% of malignancies are not identified by mammography. Negative mammogram find
should not delay ultrasound evaluation or biopsy of a clinically suspicious lesion.

Consultant Radiologist
Dr. ███
MBChB(CUHK), FRCR(UK), FHKCR, FHKAM(Radiol

病案 14
晚期子宫癌康复

2006年谭小姐四十二岁，有一名三岁的女儿。她整日忙于工作和照顾女儿，生活紧张而愉快。有一段时间她常感到小腹隐隐作痛，但并不严重，所以没有认真对待，后来又感到小腹好像较以前增大，有个包块，有时腹部胀，闭经3个月。于是她决定去看医生，经检查发现她的卵巢有个肿瘤，医生说看来是个良性肿瘤，可以用微创的方法切除，不会有大的损伤，很快就可以恢复。

脱发呕吐抗拒化疗

谭小姐于2007年8月用微创法切除了卵巢肿瘤，认为病已治好，不会再有麻烦了。没想到伤口刚刚恢复，医生就通知她需要再次进行手术，而且这次不能用微创的方法，而是要切开腹部做大型手术。原来她被切除的卵巢肿瘤经检验是恶性的，且肿瘤的来源不在卵巢在子宫，是子宫癌转移到了卵巢。癌症已发生蔓延和转移，属于晚期，需要将子宫、另侧卵巢及附件等全部清除。于是在首次术后仅一个月，于 2007 年 9 月，谭小姐再次进行了手术，切除了子宫及附件。

医生要求手术后即要做化疗。她看到许多同样的病人化疗经受了很大的痛苦，如脱发、呕吐、血细胞减低等，她心中感到害怕，不想做化疗，想试试其他的治疗方法。所以谭小姐于第二次手术后一个月，就求治于生命修复的中医药治疗。来诊时症见面色㿠白、四肢冰冷、精神疲惫、纳差食少、脉沉细涩，舌暗淡。

治则：健补脾肾，温经化瘀。

常用中药：桃仁、桂枝、白芍、茯苓、牡丹皮、鳖甲、干姜、熟地黄、当归。消瘤 2 号同时服用。

患者脾肾阳虚，积冷日久，气结经脉，致血寒积结胞宫，痞硬不消，发为癥瘕。后虽经手术切除肿瘤，但本虚标实，阳气不行，血脉凝结之主因仍然存在，况且经手术切割、缝合等，更进一步加重了经脉闭塞，气血凝滞，以及癌细胞向其他部位扩散，如不进一步治疗，原已转移的肿瘤势必复发。所用药物以温经化瘀、补肾健脾、软坚散结为主。

谭小姐按要求认真服用中药并定时去医院检查。刚开始治疗的时候，因病情严重，她每周都要来诊治，之后腹痛不适等症状逐渐减轻至消失，她就诊的时间间隔也就逐渐拉长，从一周一次到两周一次、三周一次。

谭小姐经两年左右的治疗后，已没有不适。所以她自2010年后就延长为每个月就诊一次，取药回家服用。谭小姐的状况一直良好，没有复发和转移。2011年以后，她大约隔一至两个月或两至三个月才就诊一次，服用中药也采用间断的办法，有时也会停服中药，休息一段时间。

西医难压抑癌细胞

谭小姐多年来一直都努力工作，并没有因为病重而休息过，她也没有做过化疗和放疗。从发现恶性肿瘤到现在已经十一年，她的生活和工作都保持正常。

妇科子宫、卵巢的肿瘤因位于腹部的深处，生长隐蔽，通常长到一定程度才被发现，病情一般严重难治，即使是化疗等效果也不好。这种晚期肿瘤如果说手术能够全部切除不遗留癌细胞是不大可能的，所以西医通常会进行常规化疗，效果并不理想。谭小姐术后没有进行化疗而是选择用抗癌中医药治疗，有效地控制和治疗了癌症。

诊疗记录

2007年8月27日谭小姐次右侧卵巢手术报告，腺癌来自子宫内膜。

2007年9月8日谭小姐第二次子宫切除手术报告，子宫内膜癌。

目前，谭小姐工作、生活都正常。

治癌实录 2
中晚期癌症・名家手记

附：患者检查报告

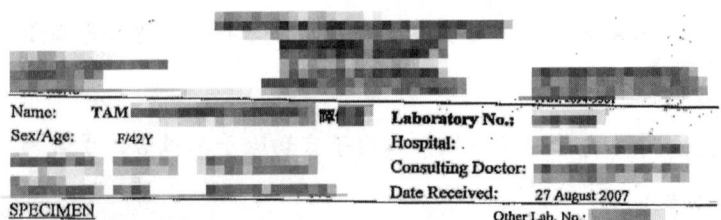

Name: TAM
Sex/Age: F/42Y
Laboratory No.:
Hospital:
Consulting Doctor:
Date Received: 27 August 2007
Other Lab. No.:

SPECIMEN
1. Right ovarian cyst.
2. Endometrial polyp and curetting.

CLINICAL SUMMARY & DIAGNOSIS
Menorrhagia, endometrial polyps.
Right ovarian cyst, ? chocolate cyst.
Laparoscopic right ovarian cystectomy, hysteroscopy, TURP and D & C.

MACROSCOPIC EXAMINATION
1. The specimen weighs 30 gm. There is an oval, previously partly opened cyst, 6 x 4.2 x 3 cm. The external surface contains moderate adhesions. The cyst wall is 0.3–1.2 cm thick and there is flat but haemorrhagic lining. There is a polypoid mural lesion, 3 x 2.2 x 1.4 cm, with a lobated yellow appearance and slightly firm cut surface. The remaining 4 fragments of tissue are consistent with cyst wall, about 2 x 2 cm in aggregate, 0.2–0.4 cm thick, with a tan smooth lining. Representative sections submitted as A1 to A3, A5 to A8 – main cyst, A4 – small fragments.

2. Multiple fragments of tan red soft tissue, 3 x 2 x 0.8 cm in aggregate. Entirely submitted as B1–B2.

MICROSCOPIC DESCRIPTION
1. Sections reveal ovarian cyst wall, partly lined by endometrial type epithelium and stroma, and partly denuded and associated with fibrosis, chronic inflammation and old haemorrhage. There is focal degenerative atypia. There are focal serosal adhesions. The nodule contains disorganized and crowded glands with complex architecture, focally forming cribriform glands, with nuclear stratification and mild to moderate nuclear atypia. Focal stromal invasion is evident, with desmoplasia and inflammation. No invasion of the subjacent cyst wall is evident and there is no involvement of the ovarian surface.

2. The endometrial fragments contain disorganized proliferative pattern endometrial glands. Many fragments are polypoid. A few fragments contain crowded back-to-back glands, some with cribriform patterns, and with stratified epithelium showing nuclear grade 1-2 features. No myometrial invasion is evident.

DIAGNOSIS
1. Right ovarian cyst
   - Endometriotic cyst, containing a 3 cm mural nodule of adenocarcinoma, endometrioid type, grade 2.
   - No invasion of cyst wall or ovarian surface involvement is evident.

2. Endometrial polyp and curetting
   - Adenocarcinoma, endometrioid type, grade 2, arising against a background of atypical complex hyperplasia.
   - No myometrial invasion is evident.

(End of report)

Date: 29 August 2007
Page: 1 of 1

MBBS(HK), MD(HK)
FHKAM(Pathology)
American Board of Pathology

MBBS(HK), MD(HK)
FHKAM(Pathology)
FRCPath(UK)

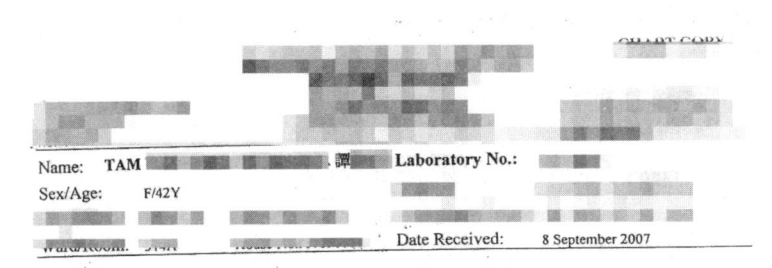

Name: TAM
Sex/Age: F/42Y
Laboratory No.:
Date Received: 8 September 2007

MICROSCOPIC DESCRIPTION
1. Sections of the upper uterine segment show focal residual complex endometrial hyperplasia with cytological atypia. These show mostly tubular glands with very focal cribriform and a back-to-back pattern. There is no residual invasive endometrioid adenocarcinoma and invasion into the myometrium is not detected. The remaining endometrium show tubular glands with proliferative activity. The cervix and upper endocervix show no additional significant pathology.
2. Sections of the right ovary show residual endometriosis with cytological atypia, consistent with atypical endometriosis. No residual adenocarcinoma is detected. There is focal tissue necrosis and fibrin deposition, consistent with previous cystectomy. The right fallopian tube shows no additional significant pathology.
3. Sections of the left ovary and left fallopian tube show no significant pathology. There is no malignancy.
4. Sections show fibroadipose tissue with focal deposition of endometrial gland and stroma, consistent with endometriosis. There is no malignancy.
5. Sections show a piece of fibromuscular tissue with no malignancy.
6. Sections show fibroadipose tissue with no malignancy.
7. Sections show fibroadipose tissue with no malignancy.
8. Sections show fibroadipose tissue and 10 lymph nodes. There is no malignancy.
9. Sections show fibroadipose tissue and 17 lymph nodes. There is no malignancy.
10. Sections show fibroadipose tissue and 6 lymph nodes. There is no malignancy.
11. Sections of the greater omentum show fibroadipose tissue. There is no malignancy.
12. Sections of the appendix show intact mucosa. There is no significant inflammation or malignancy.
13. Sections show fibrous stromal tissue with evidence of old and recent haemorrhage. Focal calcifications and foreign body granulomatous reaction are noted. There is no malignancy.

DIAGNOSIS
1. Uterus, carcinoma of endometrium, total hysterectomy
   – Residual atypical complex hyperplasia in the upper uterine segment.
   – No residual endometrioid adenocarcinoma.

2. Right ovary and right fallopian tube
   – Residual endometriosis with cytological atypia, consistent with atypical endometriosis.
   – No residual endometrioid adenocarcinoma.

3. Left ovary and left fallopian tube
   – No malignancy.

(to be continued on next page)

Date: 11 September 2007

MBBS(HK), MD(HK)
FHKAM(Pathology)
American Board of Pathology

MBBS(HK), MD(HK)
FHKAM(Pathology)
FRCPath(UK)

病案 15
末期子宫颈癌，重拾生命年华

农历立春前后，香港已是春暖花开，风景怡人。在一个天气晴朗的早晨，有一对老夫妻走进了诊所。陈先生80岁了，因患胃癌特意寻求中医药的治疗。

陈先生已进行了手术，但情况并不乐观。虽然胃的肿瘤已经切除，但手术的病理检查报告显示已经发生了较多的淋巴转移。医生也指出，这种情况一般会在术后不久发生肿瘤复发和转移，但陈先生拒绝了化疗和放疗，而特来进行抗癌中医药治疗。陪伴他求诊的陈太，今年79岁了，身腰挺直，精神饱满，气色也很好，一点也看不出是79岁的老人。她一见到医师，就赶快上前与医师握手，并急忙问道："您还认得我吗？我是您以前的病人呀！"

服药五年再无复发转移

医师看着陈太，有些迟疑，但当陈太说出她自己的姓名后，医师立刻就想起是之前熟悉的病人。她当年被癌病折磨得骨瘦如柴、虚弱难当的样子，与现在健康、满面春风的状态相比，真难想象是同一个人！大家互相问候几句后，陈太就扳起手指计算年头，原来陈太从患癌至今已有十五年了。

查找病历记录，十五年前，即2002年初，陈太六十八岁，来诊时症见四肢无力、腰膝酸软、头晕怕冷、大便坚硬，经常感到小腹收缩疼痛，虽然早已停经，但逐渐又有出血、分泌增多等异常现象，其后因病情越来越重，大腿足跟出现了多个肿块（后来才知道是肿大的淋巴结），身体越来越消瘦。脉沉细，苔白舌暗有瘀点。到医院检查，才得知她患了子宫颈癌。医生告诉她要先做化疗和放疗，然后动手术。陈太按医生的指示做了化疗和放疗，但过了一段时间后，医生说因为病情严重，即使完成所有疗程也有很大可能复发，危及生命。当时她的身体极度消瘦，每天腹痛、呕吐，头发也脱光了。陈太感到很失望，也不愿做手术了。她想，既然不能治好，就不要再去手术了。于是她来到诊所，开始用生命修复抗癌中医药治疗。

治则：温肾养肝健脾，化瘀消癥。

常用中药：鹿角片（或鹿茸）、制附子、䗪虫、大黄、蜂房、桃仁、牡丹皮、党参、黄精、枸杞子。消瘤1号同时服用。

患者年老体弱，正虚邪实，攻邪之前要顾及补正。鹿茸及鹿角片，功效相似，药力有别，根据患者病情、正气虚损程度选用，以补益肾肝、生精补血，并治腰膝痠软、崩漏带浊等症。配合制附子以补阳温通血脉，党参、黄精、枸杞子等，均为补正之药，䗪虫、大黄、蜂房均以化瘀血、破坚积为其主要功效。牡丹皮也是化脏腑癥瘕的要药，善化瘀滞而破宿癥，诸药配合，共奏扶正攻邪之功。

服用中药后陈太的病情慢慢好转，身体状态也越来越好，于是她信心大增，决心用抗癌中医药战胜癌症。她计算了一下，以抗癌中医药前后治疗五年，吃了五年的中药，起初头三年很认真吃中药，之后两年因身体没出现大问题，就间断来治疗，之后到医院检查多次，也没有什么肿瘤和异常了，她就于2007年停止了治疗。但是她仍然每年都去医院检查，而每年的检查结果都是正常的，一直没有肿瘤复发和转移。

正当平静地安度晚年之际，没想到丈夫又患了胃癌。虽然诊所已搬了地址，陈先生和陈太还是设法找到了地址。陈先生幽默地说，前些年他是配角，陪太太来治病，现在太太健康了，虽然还是跟以前一样，夫妻俩有影皆双，但现在太太是配角，他是主角，是太太陪他来用抗癌中医药治疗了。他们要互助互勉，共同战胜癌魔，共同创造长寿、健康的生活。

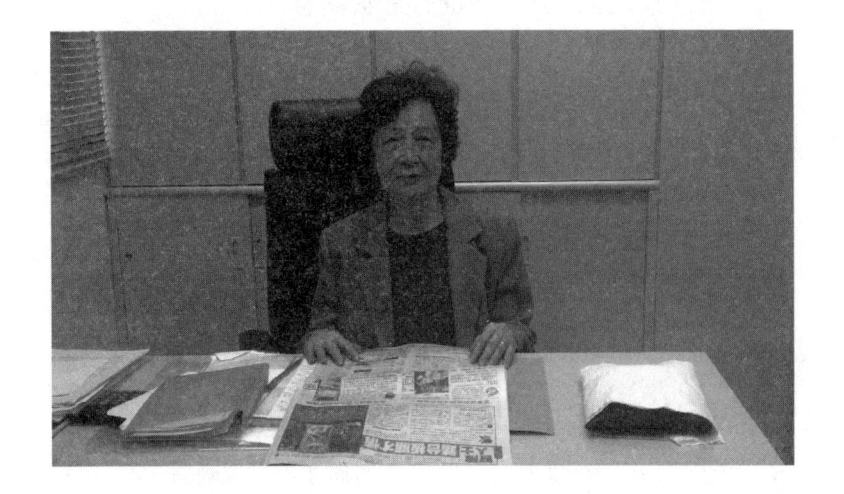

抗癌治验录 下篇

2016年6月，陈太已战胜了癌魔。

病案 16
坚持攻坚补正，战胜晚期转移癌

2005年，刘先生四十九岁，他当时有几个月常感到腰腹不适，小便颜色有些淡红，开始时他不以为意，心想可能是上火了，多饮水就会好，但其后尿色越来越不正常，直至变成血尿，他才感到可能有问题了，于是立即到医院检查，经做CT、SCAN，发现他的肾脏有个很大的肿瘤，报告上的测量显示该肿瘤竟有十厘米大。他于5月做了右肾切除手术，同月30日病理报告证实为肾细胞癌。肿瘤切除后，刘先生松一口气，心想肿瘤连同整个肾脏都已切除了，应该没有问题了。刘先生术后伤口恢复良好，心情也平静了一段时间。到2007年，他又感到不适，这次主要是咳嗽、气喘，于是又到医院检查，同年10月报告指出，发生了肾癌的肺和纵隔转移，刘先生感到很无奈，整个肾脏都已经切除了，还是转移到了肺上。于是他按西医的要求做化疗。经多方打听，刘先生得知他的病已到晚期，肺、胸膜、纵隔都有很多的转移病灶，经多次化疗后，转移病灶增大增多，化疗并没有太大的效果。

外游停药即胸痛

刘先生只好考虑用中医治疗试一试。周围的朋友说，晚期转移性多发性肿瘤，香港最好的西医医院都没办法，中医能有什么办法呢？刘先生明白如果只是一般的调理头痛脑热、跌打损伤的中医中药，肯定是治疗不了这样的重病的，但总不能坐以待毙。于是他到处寻访，下定决心找到合适的治疗方法。功夫不负有心人，刘先生终打听到生命修复抗癌中医药治疗。

来诊时刘先生身体很虚弱，气促、咳嗽、精神疲惫，化疗还造成了贫血、血细胞减少等等。随着抗癌中医药治疗，身体慢慢好转，走路活动也慢慢有了些力气。随着病情逐渐好转，刘先生感到精神好，能吃能睡，就以为没事了。长期的生病也使他精神压力很大，他想现在终于可以松一口气，外出走走了。于是他没跟任何人打招呼就外出旅游去了，两个月后才回到香港，药早就吃完了，因在旅游途中，也没有办法继续诊病和服药。回港后，他急忙到医院做检查和化验，结果显示，癌指数又升高，CT报告显示转移到双肺的肿瘤增多增大。同时又出现了胸痛、气喘的症状。

症见面色苍白、精神萎靡、胸闷、胸痛、气喘、左肺积液、咳嗽严重、连胁痛胀、吐白黏痰、食欲差、大便干结、右锁骨上质硬肿大淋巴结核桃大，舌质淡，苔白腻，脉沉弦细数。

治则：健脾疏肝益肾，散结消积。

常用中药：党参、白术、茯苓、半夏、桂枝、白芍、浙贝母、重楼、制甘遂、生大黄。

咳嗽多痰，肺郁痰盛，浊气不降，经气壅滞，胸胁痛胀，土湿胃逆，故津液不化，阴凝气闭，关窍堵塞。治宜健脾泻湿，以党参、白术、茯苓、陈皮为主，桂枝达木郁而行疏泄，白芍柔肝。制甘遂、生大黄排饮邪通下窍，浙贝母、重楼化痰，解毒散结。

医生除了给他诊病、开药之外，又耐心地对刘先生解释了治疗癌症的重要过程，由于癌症是一种恶性程度很高的特殊疾病，治疗和康复都需要很长时间，如果已经收到良好的治疗效果而中途停止用药，疾病就会反复，癌症也会卷土重来，患者本人一定要有坚定的信念，要有坚持长期治疗的思想准备和真实的行动，也需要亲人、家人的鼓励和关怀。千万不能刚好一点，症状有所改善就停止治疗。

刘先生表示以后会认真治疗不再自行中断。从此以后，刘先生以顽强的毅力与癌症抗争，每日坚持服药，如有出门，一定带上足够的中药。时从发现癌症至 2016 年随访已经有十一年多了，刘先生一直正常地生活和工作着，他今年已有五十七岁，他认为自己还年轻，还有许多事情要做，六十岁是人生的第二个青春，要更好地生活和工作。

诊疗记录

2005 年 5 月 30 日肾癌切除后，病理报告证实为肾细胞癌。

2008 年 8 月 8 日肺和胸膜转移病灶病理检查报告，证实为肾细胞癌肺转移。

2015 年 6 月，刘先生生活好，精神好。

治癌实录 2
中晚期癌症 · 名家手记

附：患者检查报告

ATIENT'S NAME		DATE RECEIVED		PATHOLOGY NO.	COPY:
LAU		30/05/2005			DR. HOSP OTHERS
.D .NO	SEX M	AGE 49 Y			
HOSPITAL	HOSPITAL NO.	CLASS		PREVIOUS PATH. NO.	

INDER CARE OF DR.

DOCTOR'S ADDRESS

CLINICAL PROCEDURE — Right nephrectomy.

CLINICAL SUMMARY — Incidental finding right kidney tumour.

FROZEN SECTION DIAGNOSIS (if any) —

PATHOLOGICAL DIAGNOSIS

Right kidney (nephrectomy)
- Grade II/III renal cell carcinoma, completely excised.

REPORT

Macroscopic examination:

Kidney within perinephric fat, 363 gms. in weight, 10 x 5.5 x 4.5 cm., partly cut-open before receipt. The renal capsule could tear off easily but was adherent to a brown-yellow firm well-defined lower pole tumour nodule 4.3 x 3.7 x 3.5 cm.

Microscopic examination:

Sections through the tumour show lobules of a renal cell carcinoma, clear cell type, with mostly only mildly pleomorphic nuclei, but some foci of moderate pleomorphism are seen with prominent nucleoli, overall amounting to a Fuhrman grade II/III tumour. Thick fibrous septa are present, and there is focal infiltration into the renal capsule, but without definite involvement of perinephric fat. No lymphovascular invasion is identified and sections of the ureteric and hilar vascular margin show no significant abnormalities. Adjacent renal parenchyma shows reactive chronic inflammation only.

Signed:

Date Reported: 31/05/2005

MBBChir(Cantab), FRCPath(UK)
FHKCPath, FHKAM(Path)

PATIENT'S NAME		DATE RECEIVED	PATHOLOGY NO.	COPY:
劉■ LAU ■■■		08/08/2008		DR. HOSP OTHERS
I.D. NO.	SEX M	AGE 52 Y		
HOSPITAL	HOSPITAL NO.	CLASS	PREVIOUS PATH. NO.	

UNDER CARE OF DR.	
DOCTOR'S ADDRESS	
CLINICAL PROCEDURE	VAT resection pleural nodules and lung nodules.
CLINICAL SUMMARY	Known CA kidney. Multiple pleural and lung metastases. VAT resection (1) pericardial nodule, (2) apical segment RLL, (3) nodules RUL, (4) nodules RLL, (5) posterior chest wall nodule and (6) nodules on diaphragm.
FROZEN SECTION DIAGNOSIS (if any)	—

PATHOLOGICAL DIAGNOSIS	(1) & (2) Pericardium and apical segment RLL (excision biopsies)
	    - Metastatic renal cell carcinoma.
	(3) RUL lung (excision biopsy) - Benign fibrosis.
	(4) to (6) Right RLL lung, posterior chest wall and diaphragm
	     (excision biopsies) - Metastatic renal cell carcinoma.

REPORT

Macroscopic examination:

(1) "Pericardial nodule" - A greyish-brown nodular piece 1.5 x 1.3 x 0.8 cm.

(2) "Apical segment right lower lobe" - A wedge-shaped lung mass 8 x 3.4 x 3.6 cm., 23.3 grams in weight. Cut surfaces showed a tan-coloured firm well-defined and solid tumour nodule 3.8 x 2.8 x 2.4 cm., 0.8 cm. from the stapled resection margin which was bulging outward and less than 0.1 cm. from the pleural surface.

(3) "Right upper lobe nodule" - A greyish-white piece 1 x 0.6 x 0.3 cm.

(4) "Right lower nodule" - A wedge-shaped brownish lung mass 4.3 x 1.4 x 1.1 cm., 2.2 grams in weight. Cut surfaces showed two light-brownish nodules 1 x 0.6 x 0.5 cm. and 0.4 x 0.3 x 0.2 cm., 0.3 cm. and 0.8 cm. from stapled resection margin and bulging outward. Also received were three tan-coloured nodular pieces 0.8 x 0.6 x 0.4 cm., 0.4 x 0.3 x 0.3 cm. and 0.3 x 0.2 x 0.1 cm.

(5) "Posterior chest wall nodule" - Four brownish pieces, largest 1.9 x 1.5 x 0.6 cm. and smallest 1.2 x 0.8 x 0.5 cm.

(6) "Nodule on diaphragm" - Thirteen greyish-brown pieces, largest 1.6 x 1.2 x 0.6 cm. and smallest 0.8 x 0.4 x 0.4 cm.

(CONTINUED ON NEXT PAGE)

Page 1 of 2

病案 17
晚期肾癌骨转移，治疗四个月可爬山

有些疼痛是治疗过程中所造成的，如放射线（放疗）所造成的纤维化组织破坏、化疗所导致的神经病变、手术所造成的组织损伤，以及手术、结扎造成的神经、血管损伤等都可引起疼痛。

双腿疼痛致行动困难

王女士（70岁）于2011年11月开始出现血尿，经检查发现肾癌，翌月接受手术切除肿瘤及右肾。手术后做放射治疗（放疗），但是在放疗四周后发现骨转移。医生又增加十次放疗，但骨转移继续加重，多处肋骨、腰椎、髋骨、盆骨、耻骨、骶骨等出现多发性骨转移，并伴有多发肺转移。骨转移是非常疼痛的，有一处骨转移就非常痛苦，王女士则有大量不同部位的骨转移。

患者疼痛难忍，服了多种止痛药和标靶药都没有作用，日夜疼痛难安。所以她于2012年10月寻求抗癌中医药治疗，当时她行动困难、双腿肿胀，不但疼痛非常剧烈，而且因为存在

多处椎骨的较大面积转移，面临瘫痪的危险。虽已使用吗啡等强力止痛药，仍疼痛剧烈。

症见表情痛苦、不停呻吟、不能站立、坐轮椅、下肢痿弱无力、进食少，舌淡红，脉细数。

治则：强骨益肾，消瘤软坚。

常用中药：熟地黄、乳香、没药、石见穿、急性子、蜈蚣、全蝎、桑寄生、威灵仙、补骨脂。消瘤丸每日3次，每次2粒，配合针灸及外用中药贴敷。

用药以抗癌、止痛、益肾、软坚、散结、消瘤为主。邪在肾，则病骨痛，为阴痹。癌性疼痛是临床治疗癌症患者最常见到的症状之一，也是令患者最痛苦的症状。使用强力镇痛药如吗啡之类非常常见，但这些止痛药只能暂时缓解疼痛或不能缓解疼痛，并且有非常多的不良反应，更有耐药性、成瘾性等严重问题，使用吗啡类的镇痛药完全出于人道主义考虑。多用于癌病无法治疗、疼痛严重不能缓解、患者又属晚期的情况。但在我们进行生命修复抗癌中医药的治疗中，患者的疼痛通常能够逐渐缓解、消失，生活质量越来越好。所以对于因疼痛而使用强力镇痛如吗啡类镇痛药的患者，需要克服成瘾性和耐药性。在服用中药的情况下，一般劝告患者逐渐减服镇痛西药，直至停用。患者一般都能配合，直到完全停止使用这些药品。

她自行停了止痛药和靶向药。三个月后，她已行动自如，4个月后甚至可以自己爬山路。现在王女士早已没有了疼痛的感觉，生活和行动都很正常，但因她的癌症有多发骨转移，多发淋巴转移和多发双肺转移，所以还在继续进行抗癌中医药治疗。

中药治疗可舒缓痛楚

用抗癌中医药治疗缓解和治愈疼痛的患者有很多。强力镇痛药是为晚期患者减少疼痛、缓解痛苦的，它对肿瘤并没有治疗作用。随着医学科学研究的发展，有效的治疗癌症的方法逐渐增多，使得患者的生活、生存的质量和时间都得以增加，就不得不考虑这些方法所带来的严重不良反应（如成瘾性）的影响。

抗癌治验录 **下篇**

诊疗记录

2011年12月17日肾癌手术切除后病理报告，证实为肾细胞癌，并已侵入淋巴、血管。

2012年5月2日MRI扫描，证实有大量多发的多部位的骨转移、双肺转移、淋巴转移。

2013年7月8日，王女士已战胜癌痛，生活正常，喜欢运动爬山。

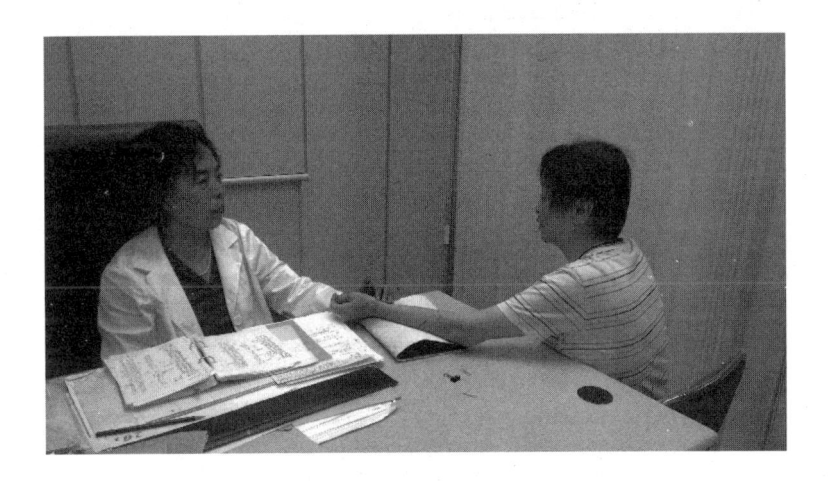

治癌实录 2
中晚期癌症 · 名家手记

附：患者检查报告

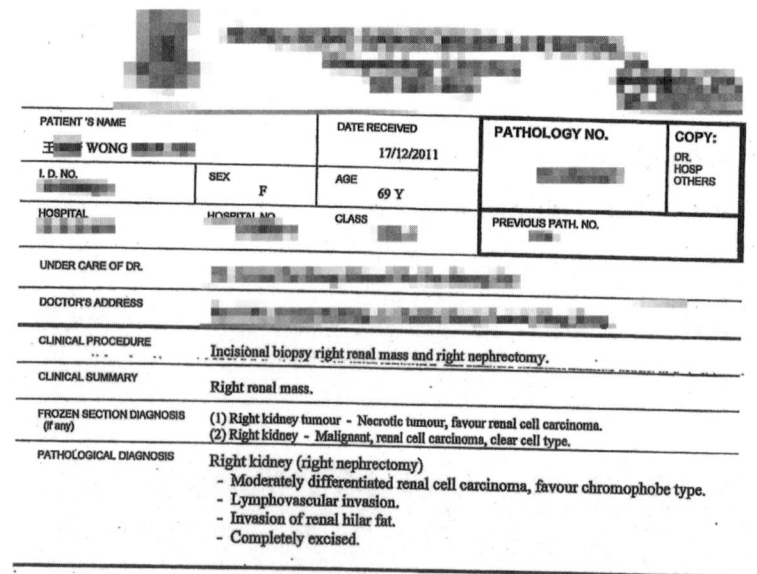

PATIENT'S NAME		DATE RECEIVED	PATHOLOGY NO.	COPY:
王 WONG		17/12/2011		DR. HOSP OTHERS
I.D. NO.	SEX F	AGE 69 Y		
HOSPITAL	HOSPITAL NO.	CLASS	PREVIOUS PATH. NO.	

UNDER CARE OF DR.	
DOCTOR'S ADDRESS	
CLINICAL PROCEDURE	Incisional biopsy right renal mass and right nephrectomy.
CLINICAL SUMMARY	Right renal mass.
FROZEN SECTION DIAGNOSIS (if any)	(1) Right kidney tumour - Necrotic tumour, favour renal cell carcinoma. (2) Right kidney - Malignant, renal cell carcinoma, clear cell type.
PATHOLOGICAL DIAGNOSIS	Right kidney (right nephrectomy) - Moderately differentiated renal cell carcinoma, favour chromophobe type. - Lymphovascular invasion. - Invasion of renal hilar fat. - Completely excised.

REPORT

Macroscopic examination:

(1) "Right kidney tumour" - Three tan pieces 1.2 x 0.8 x 0.4 cm., 0.7 x 0.6 x 0.4 cm. and 0.7 x 0.6 x 0.2 cm.

(1) "Right kidney + ureter" - Right nephrectomy specimen, 222 grams in weight, consistent with kidney 9.4 x 5 x 4.5 cm., Gerota's fascia was smooth and intact, and partial bifid ureter, joined at 10 cm. from renal hilum, total length 14 cm., upto 0.8 cm. diameter. Cut surfaces showed a yellow tan partly necrotic tumour mass 6.4 x 4 x 4 cm. occupying most of the lower and mid-pole kidney, bulging outwards coming to less than 0.1 cm. from the capsular surface. The lower pole ureter appeared dilated upto 0.7 cm. diameter, filled with yellowish necrotic tissue. The upper pole ureter was 0.4 cm. diameter, macroscopically normal. The renal capsule could tear off easily but was partly adherent to tumour.

Blocks : (A&B) tumour (C) ureteric and renovascular margin (D) hilar soft tissue
(E-J) further tumour (K) lower pole ureter (L) random kidney
(M) Gerota's fascia (N) ureter at confluence.

(CONTINUED ON NEXT PAGE)

Page 1 of 2

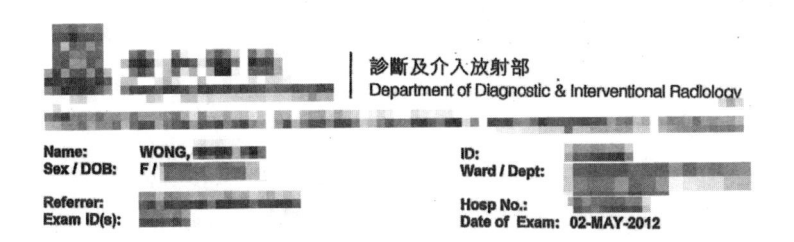

診斷及介入放射部
Department of Diagnostic & Interventional Radiology

Name: WONG, ID:
Sex / DOB: F / Ward / Dept:
Referrer: Hosp No.:
Exam ID(s): Date of Exam: 02-MAY-2012

MRI SCAN OF LEFT THIGH WITH AND WITHOUT CONTRAST

Clinical data:
Renal cell Ca. Right nephrectomy done. Completed RT to right external iliac lymph node ~ 2 months. C/o pain left upper thigh for 1 month ? cause. To assess response to RT and investigate cause of left upper thigh pain.

Technique:
Pre-contrast:
Axial T1, T2 fat sat, T1 fat saturation
Coronal T1, T2 fat sat
Sagittal T1 weighted

Post-contrast (Gadolinium):
Axial T1 fat saturation
Coronal T1 fat saturation
Sagittal T1 fat saturation

Findings:
A prominent expansile lesion is seen in the lateral part of the left superior pubic ramus. It measures 4.8 cm x 2.8 cm x 2 cm in size. It is consistent with bony metastasis. Metastatic lesion is also noted in the anterior part of the left acetabulum measuring 3.7 cm x 2.2 cm in size. Oblong-shaped area of abnormal signal is also noted in the left ischium measuring 3.1 cm x 2.2 cm in size. A metastatic mass is seen adjacent to left ischium. It measures 2.3 cm x 3.5 cm in size.
The anterior part of the left obturator internus muscle, the left obturator externus muscle, the anterior part of the left pectineus muscle, the left adductor brevis, the left adductor magnus muscle and the left quadratus femoris muscle all show increased signal on the T2-weighted fat-sat sequence and also show patchy enhancement after the IV injection of Gadolinium. They are likely due to reactive inflammatory change. No metastatic mass is actually seen in these muscles of the left upper thigh. A prominent expansile lesion is also noted in the right ilium measuring 4.4 cm x 2.3 cm in size. This is consistent with bony metastasis. No focal area of abnormal signal is noted in the left femoral head, left femoral neck or in the proximal shaft of the left femur to suggest the presence of bony metastasis. The proximal shaft of the right femur is also normal. No mass is seen in the other muscles of the left thigh to suggest metastasis. Focal area of abnormal signal is also noted in the right side of the sacrum at about S1 level. It measures 2 cm x 1.8 cm in size and is suggestive of bony metastasis. Faint area of increased signal is also noted in the right sacral ala, more inferiorly also worrisome of bony metastasis.

診斷及介入放射部
Department of Diagnostic & Interventional Radiology

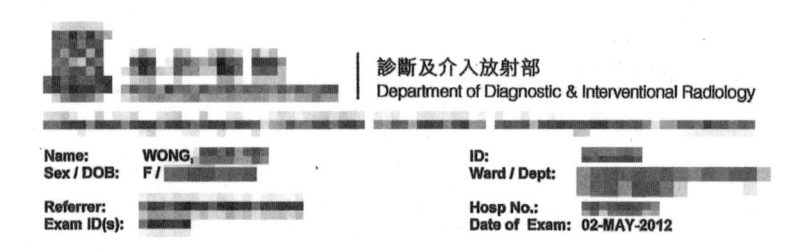

Name: WONG,
Sex / DOB: F /
Referrer:
Exam ID(s):

ID:
Ward / Dept:
Hosp No.:
Date of Exam: 02-MAY-2012

Findings: (Cont'd)
Retroperitoneum:
The right kidney is absent due to previous surgery. Several cysts are noted in the left kidney. No solid mass is seen in the left kidney. No significantly enlarged retroperitoneal lymph node is noted to suggest metastatic adenopathy. An oval-shaped T2 hyperintense mass is seen in the right side of the L3 vertebral body. It measures 3 cm x 2.9 cm in size. It is compatible with bony metastasis. A lobulated mass is also seen in the posterior element of L4 vertebra measuring 3.3 cm x 3 cm in size. It is also consistent with bony metastasis. Expansile lesion is also seen in the posterior aspect of the left 9th rib and also in the posterior aspect of the left 11th rib. They measure 2.5 cm x 2.6 cm and 4.8 cm x 3 cm in size respectively. They show enhancement after the IV injection of Gadolinium and are consistent with bony metastases. Incidentally noted are multiple nodules in both lung bases worrisome of pulmonary metastases.

Pelvis:
Uterus is not enlarged. No obvious focal uterine mass is seen. Both ovaries are also not enlarged. An oval shaped right common iliac node is noted, measuring 2.1 cm x 1.5 cm in size, likely deu to residual metastatic adenopathy. Metastatic lesion is seen in the right ilium measuring 4.4 cm x 2.3 cm in size. Metastatic lesion is also noted in the left ischium measuring 3.1 cm x 2.2 cm in size. A metastatic mass is also seen adjacent to left ischium measuring 2.3 cm x 3.5 cm in size. Prominent metastatic lesion is seen in the left anterior acetabulum measuring 3.7 cm x 2.2 cm in size. Metastatic lesion is also noted in the lateral superior pubic ramus associated with a metastatic mass. It measures 4.8 cm x 2.8 cm x 2 cm in size. Metastatic lesion is also noted in the right side of the sacral ala.

診斷及介入放射部
Department of Diagnostic & Interventional Radiology

Name: WONG,
Sex / DOB: F /
Referrer:
Exam ID(s):

ID:
Ward / Dept:
Hosp No.:
Date of Exam: 02-MAY-2012

Impression:
1. Metastatic lesions are seen in the left 9th rib, left 11th rib, the right side of the L3 vertebral body, the posterior element of the L4 vertebra, right ilium, left ischium, left acetabulum and the lateral part of right superior pubic ramus. Metastatic lesion is also noted in the right side of the sacral ala.

2. Two hemangioma are noted in the right lobe of liver.

3. Evidence of previous right nephrectomy is noted.

4. Multiple nodules are noted in both lower lobes worrisome of pulmonary metastases.

5. Residual right common iliac adenopathy is noted, measuring 2.1 cm x 1.5 cm in size

Department of Diagnostic & Interventional Radiology
MBBS FRCR FHKCR FHKAM(Radiology)

Typed By:

Approved Date-Time:
02-MAY-2012 07:17 PM

Received at _____ Time _____ Read by Dr. _____ Signature _____ Date _____ Time _____
         dd/mm/yy   dd/mm/yy

病案 18
晚期癌症创奇迹，勇征喜马拉雅山

李小姐喜欢旅行，经常在为下一次旅程做准备，生活充满期待及色彩。生活规律正常的她，闲时都会跟朋友聚会，分享生活趣事，偶然有小病，很快就可痊愈。可是，1993年，李小姐常感到下腹阵痛，持续时间相当长，医生都查不出原因，家人认为小心为上，因此要求她去做详细检查。检查报告指出她患了肾癌，这对当时四十七岁的她来说很难接受，认为生活健康的自己怎么可能患上这种绝症！

发现肺肿瘤

庆幸有家人的支持和安慰，她努力接受了这个事实，也明白消极是起不了作用的，惟有积极面对才能战胜病魔，因此她找了最好的医院和医生切除了整个右肾，当时肿瘤有十厘米大，医生说，整个都切除了，周围也清理得很干净，应该不需要担心了。

但是几年后，她逐渐感到体力不如从前，其后又出现气促、咳嗽、胸闷等症状。在2004年检查时发现肺转移，且肺的转移肿瘤为多发性，肿瘤遍布双肺的各个部位，并导致呼吸困难、咯血、胸痛，医生告知，已无法可医，生命垂危。

李小姐对这个结果表示很不甘心，她问医生，为什么别的癌症患者可以做化疗和放疗，她就不可以试试？医生回答说，当然可以试，但是肾癌晚期发生多发性大面积肺转移者，化疗和放疗并无效果，而且会造成身体更加虚弱衰竭，导致生命更快结束。

服用中药后有好转

事实上，李小姐本人也是抗拒放疗和化疗的，因为她明白其伤害性很大。现在她更明白连化疗和放疗都被直接告知没用。有一天李小姐从朋友得知生命修复抗癌中医药治疗的效果很好。经朋友介绍，她前来求治。在她认知里，中医功效较慢，她怀疑自己能等得及吗？毕竟，癌细胞已大量转移到肺了。

来诊时，症见疲乏无力，气短难续，咳嗽胸闷，腰痛腿软，失眠纳差，舌淡，脉沉细数。

治则：补阴护阳，肺肾双治。

常用中药：浙贝母、重楼、蜂房、百合、龟甲胶、肉苁蓉、石见穿、天南星、半夏、山药、沙参。散结丸、消瘤粉同时服用。

贝母、半夏、百合、蜂房、重楼、石见穿等针对多发性双肺转移，有止咳、化痰散结、抗癌之效，肉苁蓉、龟甲胶、沙参等益肺补肾，调整阴阳，以达"阴平阳秘，精神乃治"。

肺为娇脏，易受邪侵，肺部有大量转移性肿瘤更需长期精心调治，方可使病情逐趋好转，肺肾双治，还须常常顾及脾胃中土，土可生金。

家人都劝李小姐积极治疗，服药也应持之以恒。这期间，她耐心地听从吩咐：定时服药、敷药，从不间断。经过多月治疗，她的身体状况有了明显改善，之前咳嗽、咯血、呼吸困难、失眠等症状均已逐渐减轻，癌指数也降低了。到2006年，她已经能够正常生活，周围的人和朋友没人能想到她是晚期癌症患者。

李小姐用抗癌中医药治疗已有多年，肺部的大量多发性肿瘤逐渐稳定、缩小，也没有再出现新的病灶。她仍然经常和朋友一起出门旅游，欣赏大自然的美景，也为了了解自己的身体能否承受更多的挑战。

2011年夏天，李小姐更去了喜马拉雅山旅游。攀登这座举世闻名的最高雪山是她年轻时的梦想。患了癌症之后，李小姐以为此生都无法实现这个愿望了。可是，连她自己也没有料到，在她年老之后，患有晚期癌症之时，不但攀登上了喜马拉雅山，而且还登上了海拔五千米高处的大本营。她用顽强的生命创造了人间奇迹。

患癌至今已有二十四年

当李小姐从世界之巅喜马拉雅山返回香港，又去诊所就诊时，她是那么轻松又那么随便地告诉我们，身体和内心的感受都非常好。她以六十六岁的年龄、晚期癌症的身体登上了喜马拉雅山海拔五千米的大本营，我由衷地为她高兴，同时计算了一下李小姐从患癌症至今已有二十年了。

有人可能不相信，认为是诊断有错。但是李小姐长期的病历以及每年的检查报告，包括肺转移以后的病理检查报告等，都在完好地保存着，随时可以拿出来进行严格的医学鉴定。通过这些真实案例，更加证明了癌症不是绝症，癌症是能够被人类征服的。

诊疗记录

1993年3月8日肾癌手术切除后，病理报告证实为肾腺癌。

2007年10月23日CT检查报告证实有双肺和胸膜大量多发癌转移病灶。

2011年8月，李小姐击退癌魔后，登上景色优美的喜马拉雅山圆梦。又过了五年多了，李小姐仍然经常旅游和运动，生活充满乐趣。

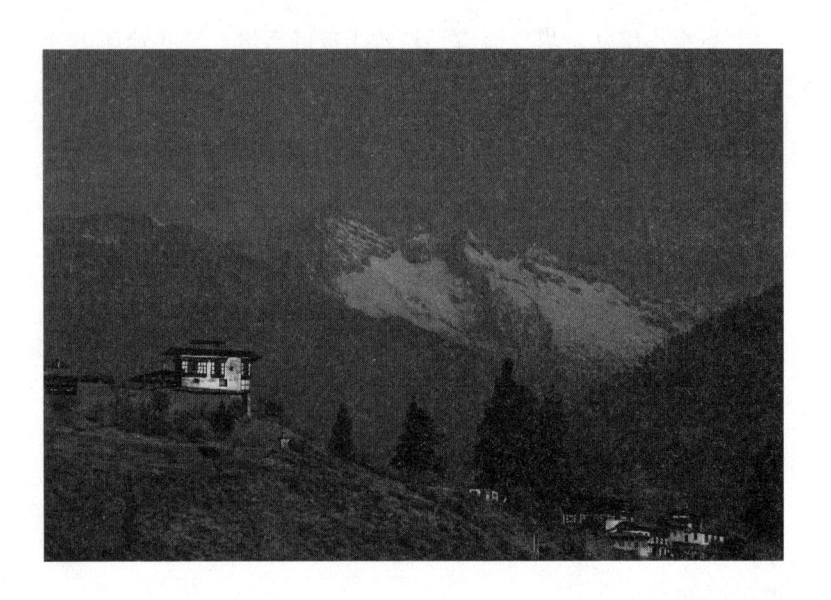

抗癌治验录 下篇

附：患者检查报告

HISTOPATHOLOGY REPORT

Pathology No. _____
Previous Path. No. _____

Name: LEE _____ I.D. No. _____ Sex/Age: F/47 Date received: 8-3-93 (20:55)
Hosp. or O.P.D. No _____ Ward/Bed No. 735 (1) Doctor _____
Specimen: Rt. kidney

Clinical summary/diagnosis
RUQ pain
Ultrasound & CT showed large tumour in Rt. kidney
Rt. radical nephrectomy done

GROSS DESCRIPTION
The specimen consists of a right nephrectomy weighing 438 gm. The kidney measures 13.5 cm. superior-inferiorly, 9 cm. medio-laterally and 7.5 cm. antero-posteriorly. It is surrounded by some fat. The attached ureter is 4 cm. in length. On sectioning, a large oval tumour is situated in the upper pole measuring 10 cm. at its greatest diameter. The cut surface of the tumour is yellowish with extensive haemorrhagic as well as microcystic degeneration. The tumour extends into the upper calyx dilating it. Some blood is seen in the lower calyx which is normal sized. No obvious tumour are seen in branches of the renal vein.
- (A) Transverse section of the ureter.
- (B) & (C) Represent one plane of sections taken from the hilum of the kidney.
- (B) Contain the tumour protrusion into the upper calyx.
- (C) Includes the renal vein.
- (D), (E), (F) & (G) Representative section of the tumour with (G) including the capsule.
- (H) Additional section of the hilum.
- (I) Represents the normal-looking kidney.

MICROSCOPIC DESCRIPTION
Section of the solid yellowish nodule in the centre of the lesion shows atypical cells with large hyperchromatic vesicular nuclei and prominent nucleoli. The cytoplasm is moderate and is either clear or amphophilic. These cells form small clusters and tubular structures surrounded by delicate fibrovascular stroma. This central solid nodule is surrounded by large cysts lined by cells with minimally enlarged and slightly hyperchromatic vesicular nuclei surrounded by abundant pinkish granular cytoplasm resembling oncocytes. The lumen of these cysts contains abundant proteinaceous material admixed with blood and has a microcystic appearance on gross-examination. The features are that of adenocarcinoma of the kidney (hypernephroma). The renal vessels at the hilum contain no tumour. The tumour is confined within the kidney. The capsule has not been penetrated. The rest of the renal calyx and pelvis shows mild chronic non-specific inflammation. Section of the ureter is unremarkable.

DIAGNOSIS
Nephrectomy (right) - Adenocarcinoma of the kidney.
- Tumour confined within the kidney with no invasion of renal vein.
- T_2, N_x, M_x.
Assuming there is no lymph node and distant metastasis, this is stage II.

DATE _____ 10.3.93

```
04-09-28 05:56 PM                    HISTOPATHOLOGY                              H 1
```

PATIENT'S NAME		DATE RECEIVED	PATHOLOGY NO.	COPY:
李██ LEE ██████		16/09/2004	██████	DR. HOSP OTHERS
I.D.NO	SEX F	AGE 58 Y		
HOSPITAL	HOSPITAL NO.	CLASS	PREVIOUS PATH. NO.	

UNDER CARE OF DR.

DOCTOR'S ADDRESS

CLINICAL PROCEDURE Core biopsies of 8 mm. nodule.

CLINICAL SUMMARY Carcinoma of kidney. Three small nodules 0.5 - 0.8 cm. in diameters.

FROZEN SECTION DIAGNOSIS (if any)

PATHOLOGICAL DIAGNOSIS

Lung (core biopsy) - Secondary adenocarcinoma.

REPORT

Supplementary Report

Immunohistochemical studies show the tumour cells are negative for TTF-1 (lung and thyroid), CK7 and CK20. The results would be more consistent with secondary adenocarcinoma from kidney, as diagnosed.

Name: LEE,
Sex/Age/DOB: F/62
Ref.Dr.:
Exam ID.:

ID No.:
Room/Bed: /
Hospital No.:
Date of Exam: 23 Oct, 2007

LOW DOSE CT SCAN OF THORAX

Clinical data:
Ca kidney.

Technique:
One AP scout. 5 mm thick slices at 5 mm intervals through the thorax using low dose technique.

Findings:
Nodules of variable size are seen in the lungs. Their size and distribution are as follows:
1. R upper lobe, anterior subpleural region (0.28x0.22cm).
2. R middle lobe, medial aspect (0.56x0.22cm).
3. R middle lobe, anterior subpleural (0.39x0.28cm).
4. R lower lobe, medial aspect of posterior costophrenic sulcus (0.72x0.66cm).
5. R lower lobe, posterior (0.68x0.69cm).
6. L lower lobe, posterior (0.37x0.37cm).
7. L upper lobe, anterior (0.74x0.49cm).
8. L upper lobe, medial aspect (0.37x0.68cm).
9. L upper lobe, anterior subpleural (0.19x0.19cm).
10. L upper lobe, lingula (1.27x1.27cm).
11. L lower lobe, posterolateral subpleural (0.39x0.35cm).
12. L lower lobe, posterolateral subpleural (0.39x0.36cm).
13. L lower lobe, posterior subpleural (0.31x0.37cm).
14. L lower lobe, posterior subpleural (1.12x1.06cm).
For those that are tiny in size and subpleural in location, they are radiologically nonspecific.
For those that are bigger in size, given the clinical history of this patient, findings are suggestive of lung secondaries.

Two calcified granuloma are seen. The one seen in posterior subpleural region of L upper lobe measures 0.28cm in size. The one seen in apical segment of L lower lobe measures 0.17cm in size.

Mediastinum is clear. No lymphadenopathy is noted.

Hila appear unremarkable.

Imaged portion of liver and adrenals appear unremarkable.

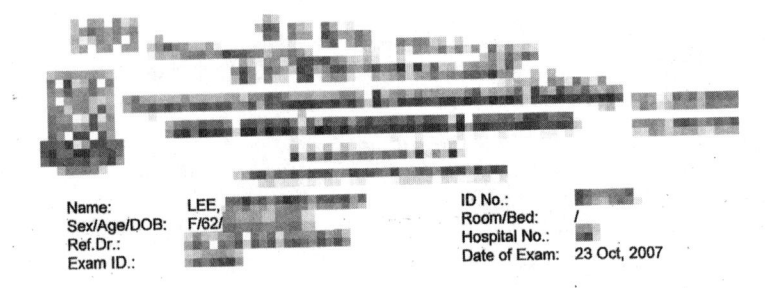

治癌实录 2
中晚期癌症・名家手记

Name: LEE,
Sex/Age/DOB: F/62/
Ref.Dr.:
Exam ID.:

ID No.:
Room/Bed: /
Hospital No.:
Date of Exam: 23 Oct, 2007

Impression:
1. Comparison is made with last low dose CT scan of thorax dated 27 Jul. 2007.

2. Multiple lung secondaries with extent as aforesaid. (N.B.: For those nodules that are tiny in size and subpleural in location, they are radiologically nonspecific.)

3. Two sizeable lung secondaries have mild interval increase in size:
a. L upper lobe, lingula
This now measures 1.27x1.27cm in size (last time, it measured 1.25x1.22cm in size).
b. L lower lobe, posterior subpleural
This now measures 1.12x1.06cm in size (last time, it measured 1.0x0.82cm in size).

4. The rest of the small lung secondaries show no significant interval change in size. No new lung secondary is noted.

MBBS(HK) FRCR(UK) FHKCR FHKAM(Radiology)

TRANSCRIBED BY: SARETA

病案 19
两种恶癌集一身，抗癌疗法显奇功

邝先生，八十二岁，于 2007 年初开始出现小便频繁、腹痛、小便时疼痛、疲乏无力等症状。他去医院检查发现前列腺有肿瘤，于是按医院的安排做了放疗和化疗。之后又发生咳嗽，并且越咳越严重。他再次去医院做进一步检查才发现原发肿瘤在膀胱。他患了膀胱癌，并且是最晚期，已经发生前列腺的侵入和转移，而且恶性程度很高，病情非常严重，医院认为无法再医。

祸不单行，邝先生除了膀胱和前列腺的肿瘤无法治疗外，咳嗽还越来越重，并发展到咯血。医院安排他于 2007 年 4 月做了 PET-CT 检查，发现双肺都有许多肿瘤。肺脏的肿瘤也是由膀胱癌转移而来吗？或是另有其他原因？

为诊断清楚，他于 2007 年 4 月 26 日又做了肺的活组织检查，结果病理诊断为非小细胞性肺癌。这是与膀胱癌完全不同的肿瘤，是来源于肺的癌症。就是说，邝先生患了原发性的非小细胞性肺癌，并有广泛的双肺转移，同时又患了膀胱癌，并已经侵入到前列腺。

恶性肿瘤转移扩散

患一种癌症已是大难临头,多少人经全力救治也无希望。邝先生是患了两种恶性肿瘤,而且两种癌症均已发生了转移和扩散,也同是晚期。

他当时病情危险,百般无奈下,求治于生命修复抗癌中医药治疗。来诊时症见咳嗽、呼吸困难、气喘、咯血、头晕无力、腹痛、尿痛、小便困难、血尿、极度虚弱,舌淡,脉浮细无力。

治则:健脾益肾。

常用中药:人参、茯苓、山药、熟地黄、天冬、桑螵蛸、黄精、贝母、杏仁、王不留行、猪苓、穿山甲、急性子、石见穿。散结粉同时服用。

熟地黄、天冬、桑螵蛸、黄精补益脾肾。贝母、杏仁、王不留行、猪苓、穿山甲利湿散结通络。急性子、石见穿健脾抗癌。患者年老体衰,加上集两种癌(肺癌、肾癌)于一身,健脾益肾是统治全身之法。除补益先后天之本,还须攻积消瘤,如急性子、石见穿等都是抗癌的有效中药。

按照常规,邝先生这种情况早该放弃治疗了。但医生和病人都坚持治疗，不愿放弃，终于出现了奇迹。经过治疗，邝先生的精神状态逐渐改善，咳嗽逐渐减少，小便也逐渐好转了。

邝先生认为已无大碍，所以于 2008 年停止了抗癌中医药治疗。不料没多久，许多的严重症状又再次出现，咳嗽严重到不能睡眠，还有尿痛、腹胀痛等。邝先生于是再来就诊，表示要认真治疗。又经过约两年的抗癌中医药治疗，他的健康才基本恢复正常，没有严重咳嗽、气喘，大小便也基本正常。此后邝先生仍断续到诊所调理身体，生活已完全恢复正常。

如今邝先生八十二岁了，生活可以自理，患上感冒等病也会及时来诊，在调理身体的同时也常用中药进行持续的抗癌治疗。他说这些年再也没去过医院。现在已整整六年过去了，从当初严重的病情逐渐得到缓解到目前生活正常，证实了抗癌中医药治疗晚期肿瘤多发转移是有效的。

六年治疗病情稳定

邝先生精神饱满，自己可以料理日常生活，他说，自己去过一次鬼门关又回来了，现在要珍惜晚年得之不易的生活，继续调理身体，继续用抗癌中医药治疗。

患两种恶性肿瘤者较为少见，而两种均为晚期、均有转移的患者病情更危险。本例患者经过病理活组织检查，证实为两种原发性的恶性肿瘤，且均已发生转移。这样严重的病情，仅用抗癌中医药治疗就能够使病情长期稳定，患者生活正常，说明中医药是能够有效抗癌的。尤其是当患者自以为病情无大碍而停止服中药后，病情就会明显反复，更说明了中医药有效的治疗作用。至2013年，家人再次安排邝先生去接受西医治疗，故失访。

2013年初邝先生患两种恶性肿瘤，仍然生活正常。

诊疗记录

2007年5月26日主诊医生的病情介绍，证实患上晚期膀胱癌侵入前列腺，以及患有非小细胞肺癌伴多发肺转移。

抗癌治验录 下篇

附：患者检查报告

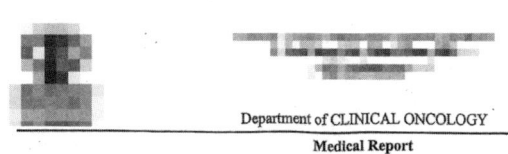

Department of CLINICAL ONCOLOGY

Medical Report

Date: 26/05/2007

To whom it may concern

Name: KWONG,
Sex: Male
Date of Birth: 1931
HKID:
Our Ref:

Mr. KWONG, has past medical history of hypertension and essential thrombocythaemia. He is on hydroxyurea since 2004.

He presented with prostatism and haematuria since December, 2006.
Cystoscopy was performed in Pamela Youde Nethersole Eastern Hospital/ Surgery on 12/1/07 and showed Intravesical prostatic extension, making examination of bladder base and ureteric orifice difficult. Intravenous urogram showed no significant lower urinary tract obstruction. He was given Proscar for management of prostatism.

Mr Kwong consulted private urologist for TURP. Cystoscopy on 15/3/07 showed suspicious sessile growth over trigone obscuring the right ureteric orifice and infiltrating the prostate causing obstruction. Resection of tumour was done. Pathology showed poorly differentiated urothelial cell carcinoma with involvement of prostate gland.

PET-CT in 4/2007 showed multiple hypometabolic lung nodules, with another hot nodules of 2.2cm (SUV 5.7) in LLZ. No other regional or distant secondaries.

CT guided biopsy of left upper lobe lung mass was performed on 26/4/2007. Pathology is highly suspicious of non-small cell carcinoma of lung.

In summary, the patient suffers from double primary including carcinoma of bladder with invasion to prostate
and non-small cell carcinoma of lung with multiple lung metastasis.

He is now on palliative chemotherapy Gemzar/ carboplatin.

This statement is true to the best of my knowledge and belief.

Signature:

Page 1 of 2

病案 20
击退癌魔，笔端生辉

2007年初，63岁的麦女士皮肤开始发硬、发痒，她以为自己跟其他老人家一样，只是因为皮肤保湿功能不好加上饮食不佳所致。因此她除了觉得瘙痒不便之外并不特别担心。但随着日子一天天过去，疼痛和瘙痒处越来越多，范围也越来越大，什么止痒膏药、解痒丸散也不奏效。后来皮肤迅速溃烂，越来越痛，她才去求医。

医生看她左臀大片溃烂的皮肤，觉得非同小可，要求她尽快做活组织的病理检查。医生的神情令她担心，她也不敢怠慢，赶忙通知女儿陪她到医院做检查。

淋巴转移，腹剧痛失眠

在等待检查结果期间，女儿对母亲发出善意的责怪，怪她不早日跟亲人沟通。麦女士也承认是自己过分大意、乱用成药、自误医期，皮肤没治好却将肠胃拖垮了，以致时常腹痛。

结果，麦女士被院方确诊为皮脂腺癌。院方建议在进行手术切除前，先用计算机扫描以确定癌症病变范围。全身检查结果更出人意料，原来麦女士经常腹痛并不是因为乱服成药弄坏肠胃那么简单，而是由于已有多发性的腹腔淋巴结转移。

医生决定先做手术切除臀部大面积的皮肤。2007年4月10日，手术非常成功，愈合情况良好。可是麦女士仍腹痛不止，大腿足跟亦出现硬结和肿块。院方于是又为她做了计算机扫描，检验结果显示，她不但有腹部淋巴转移，而且还有肠系膜和腹股沟等多处淋巴转移，医院确诊为癌症第四期，即最晚期。

接受了医院安排化疗后，她的病情还是没有改善，不能如常进食，并且有腹痛、失眠、咳嗽带血及淋巴结肿大。由于病情已是晚期，西医药已没有治疗的办法和希望了。

因此，麦女士于2007年6月开始接受生命修复抗癌中医药治疗，当时她疲态毕露，精神状态很差，失眠，下腹部及腹股沟有可触及的多个肿瘤且疼痛胀满。腹部胀满疼痛，双腿肿胀麻木，腹股沟处疼痛，腰背痠痛，舌淡，脉沉。

治则：除湿解毒，软坚散结。

常用中药：土茯苓、白鲜皮、生薏苡仁、蜈蚣、全蝎、乳香、没药、白芥子、海藻、昆布。散结丸同时服用。

土茯苓、生薏苡仁解毒除湿走表，乳香、没药、白芥子，散结软坚。

其后的两年，麦女士专心用抗癌中医药治疗。肿大的淋巴结逐渐消失，肿瘤也逐渐消失。她继续坚持服用中药，肿瘤消失了，精神状态焕然一新。她同时也开始了新的生活，学习书法、字画，锻炼身体，旅游，打乒乓球，料理大量家务。

十年过去，麦女士现已七十四岁，她说，以前得了癌症很伤心，每天的日子都很痛苦，现在感到比以前更年轻有劲，全靠抗癌中医药治疗救了命。她还不能离开这个世界，她的责任和工作还没有完成，家中上有老，下有小，全靠她照料。这三位老人，一是家婆，已经九十多岁了，不能没有她的照顾；第二个是她自己；第三个是她的狗，已经养了十多年，按人寿命比例，已是九十多岁了，也需要她照顾。她还有儿有女，一家人她全要负起责任。她现在很开心，表示生活的重担压不垮她，并且要告诉大家她叫麦翠屏。

强烈日照诱发皮肤癌

长期持续的强烈日光照射是皮肤癌的诱发因素之一。化学致癌物如芳香烃、煤焦油等也是公认的致癌物质。在皮肤癌患者中,从事放射工作者较常见。此外,烧伤和外伤后慢性骨髓炎的引流窦道并发引起的皮肤癌也可见到。

抗癌中医药治疗中扶正祛邪、散结解毒的方法,对于控制并逐渐缩小癌变皮肤和癌性溃疡范围、止痛、提高免疫功能等都有良好效果。

诊疗记录

麦女士,63岁,皮肤癌淋巴转移。

2007年4月25日同位素及正电子扫描部报告证实:左腹股沟区有大量转移性淋巴结肿瘤,腹部有大量转移性肠系膜淋巴结肿瘤。

2017年2月麦女士接受抗癌中医药诊治后成功击退癌魔。

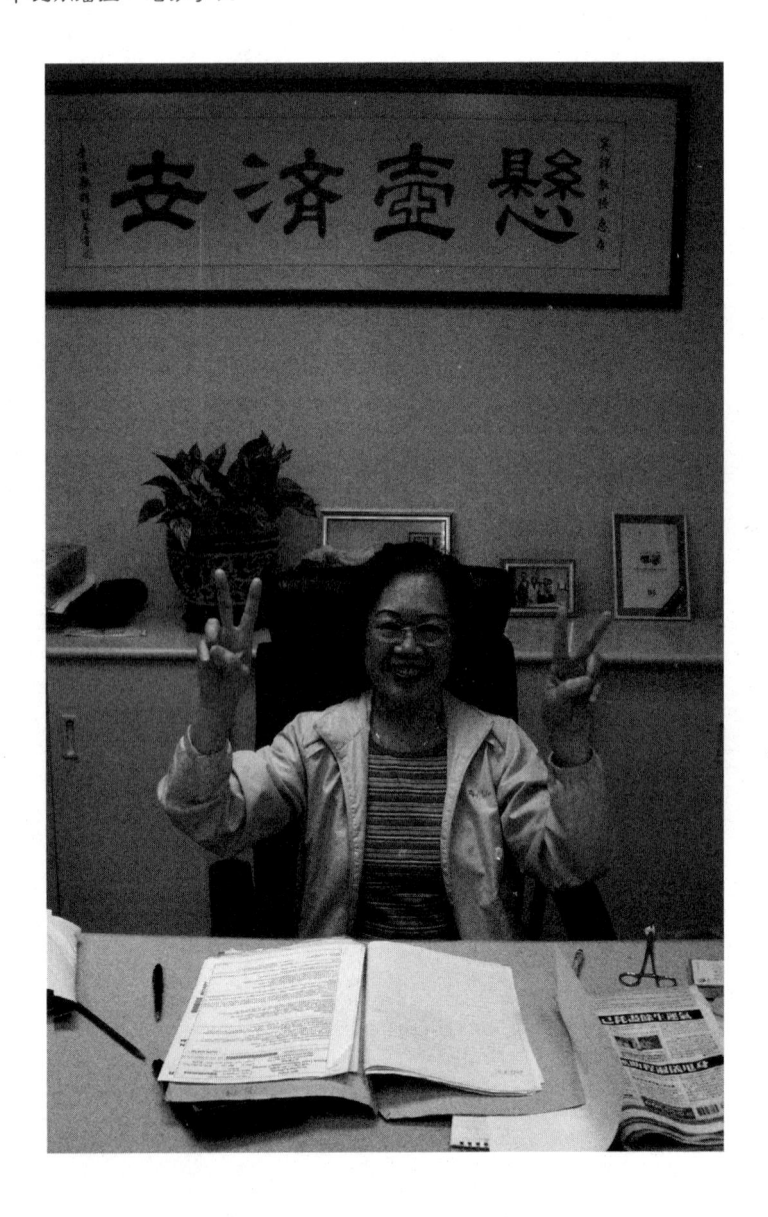

治癌实录 2
中晚期癌症·名家手记

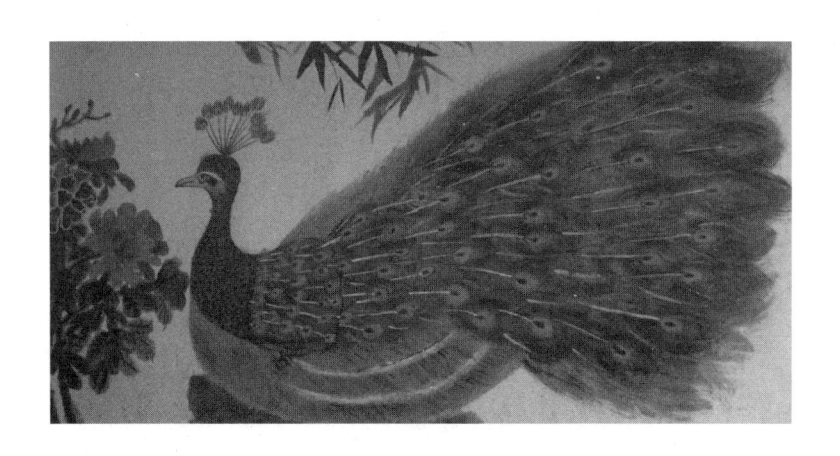

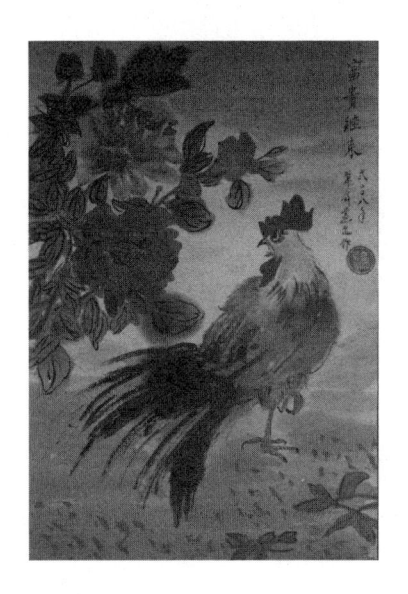

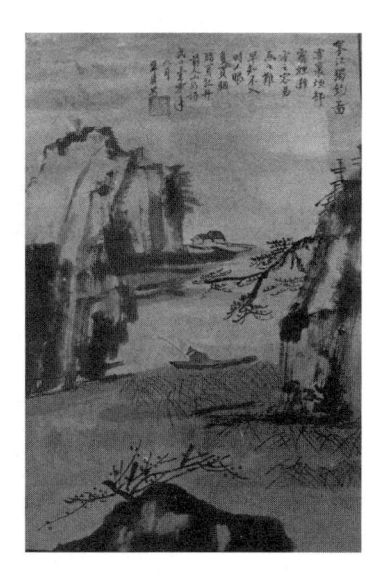

抗癌治验录 下篇

治癌实录 2
中晚期癌症·名家手记

附：患者检查报告

醫院 同位素及正電子掃描部
Department of Nuclear Medicine & Positron Emission Tomography
HOSPITAL

Name:	Mak,		Date:	25/4/2007
I.D. No.:	A11	Sex:	Female	
Hosp. No.:		Age:	63 Y	Fax:
Ward/Dept.:				Tel:

POSITRON EMISSION TOMOGRAPHY
(^{18}F-FDG ONCOLOGY)

<u>History:</u>

A 63 year-old lady initially presented with 2 left groin masses. She was diagnosed sebaceous carcinoma of left buttock with excision done on 10/4/2007. One left groin node was excised and confirmed lymph node metastasis. Pre-operative CT scan showed a cluster of enlarged mesenteric lymph nodes up to 2.5 cm in lower abdomen and suspected of metastasis. PET scan for further investigation. DM on oral medication. No history of hepatitis or tuberculosis.

<u>Radiopharmaceutical:</u> 10.8 mCi F-18 Fluorodeoxyglucose (^{18}FDG) injected intravenously.

<u>Findings:</u>

Limited whole body CT transmission and PET emission imaging began at 46 minutes after radiopharmaceutical administration (blood glucose 6.8 mmol/l), spanning a region from vertex to toe. 60 mg Spasmonal was given p.o. 15 min before ^{18}FDG administration.

Liver tissue normal reference uptake has a SUVmax of 3.65 and delayed SUVmax of 2.66.

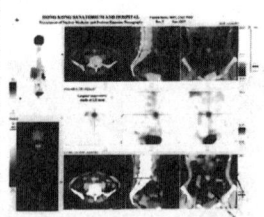

There are diffuse mild activities in the medial left groin and left buttock regions and likely represent post-operative inflammatory changes. A focally hypermetabolic left groin node is seen more laterally. The right groin appears normal with no abnormal lymphadenopathy. In addition, multiple enlarged hypermetabolic mesenteric nodes are identified in the lower abdomen with the largest one noted at L5 level. These are most consistent with multiple metastatic mesenteric lymphadenopathy. There is no abnormal uptake in the uterine and bilateral adnexal regions. The liver shows uniform uptake without any focal area of hypermetabolism. The adrenal glands and pancreas appear normal. The bowel shows some physiological activity. There is no hypermetabolic intramammary lesion in the breasts. Both lungs reveal no focal abnormal glycolysis. The mediastinum and bilateral hila show normal physiological activities. Bilateral supraclavicular and cervical lymph nodes are unremarkable. There is no abnormal uptake in the nasopharynx. Marrow activities within the axial skeleton are normal. No other suspicious hypermetabolic skin lesion is noted in the remaining regions of the body.

Functional parameters of these lesions are tabulated below:

Mak, Chui Ping				Standard	Delayed
Site	X	Y	Z	SUVmax	SUVmax
Liver (normal)				3.65	2.66
Largest mesenteric node at L5 level	1.9	2.4	2.0	3.81	6.57
Mesenteric node at S1 level	1.3	1.2	1.2	3.20	3.10
Lt groin node	1.0	1.2	1.0	2.52	2.92
Lt buttock activity	2.4	2.8	2.5	1.62	1.95

<u>Impression:</u>

1. Multiple metastatic lymphadenopathy are identified as left groin node and multiple mesenteric nodes in the lower abdomen.
2. Post-operative inflammatory changes in the left buttock and medial left groin regions.
3. No other metabolic evidence of solid organ involvement is noted.

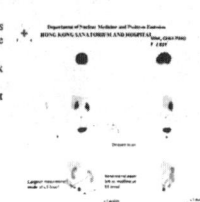

MBBS(HK), FRCR, FHKAM (Radiology)
Specialist in Nuclear Medicine, Department of Nuclear Medicine & P.E.T., HKSH

抗癌治验录 下篇

醫院 同位素及正電子掃描部
Department of Nuclear Medicine & Positron Emission Tomography
HOSPITAL

Name: Mak,
I.D. No.: A1
Hosp. No.:
Ward/Dept.:

Sex: Female
Age: 63 Y

Date: 3/8/2007
Ref. Dr.:
Fax:
Tel:

Impression:

1. Resolved mesenteric and left groin nodal metastases. As understood, metabolic quiescence is not equivalent to true tumoricidal effect. At least 2 serial PET studies demonstrating no abnormal metabolism may be considered more confirmative of metabolic remission.
2. Resolved previous post-operative inflammatory changes in the left groin and left buttock activity.
3. No new lesion is seen.

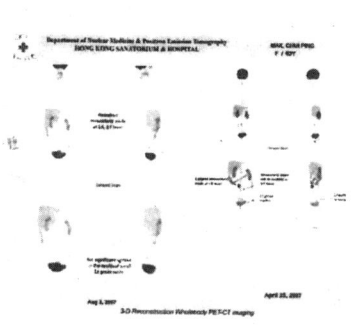

_____, MBBS(HK), FHKCR, FHKAM (Radiology)
Specialist in Nuclear Medicine, Department of Nuclear Medicine & P.E.T., HKSH

病案 21
攻坚通络，消散大量肿瘤兼腹水

腹部是人体的重要部位，也是最容易发生病变的部位。许多重要的脏器都在腹部，例如肝、脾、胆、胃、肾、肾上腺、小肠、大肠、胰、膀胱、尿道、子宫等等，包括了消化系统、泌尿系统、生殖系统，还有一些内分泌系统等。如果腹部患恶性肿瘤，危害很大。肿瘤会影响到相关器官的正常生理功能，也容易发生腹水、水肿，并进一步导致全身各器官功能衰竭。常见的肝癌、胃癌、胰腺癌等都会出现这种情况。腹部有很多脏器，如果一个器官的恶性瘤转移到附近脏器，则使疾病影响范围扩大，使得受累器官也发生病变和功能障碍。

如果肿瘤在腹腔内广泛扩散转移则后果更为严重。汤女士就是这种情况。她患有卵巢癌，之后不但转移到两侧卵巢等生殖系统，更转移到肝、脾、肾、肾上腺、肠等很多脏器。

2009年，汤女士42岁，常感腹部疼痛不适、腹部增大。其后发生气喘、呼吸困难，腹部越来越大，她于2010年1月到医院检查，结果为卵巢癌晚期广泛转移，检查报告指出，她的盆腔和腹腔中有很多大肿瘤，并伴有肝肾转移，肝下方肿瘤为

14.5cm×12.3cm×12.7cm，左肾区肿瘤 6cm×6cm×6.6cm，肝门位肿瘤 5.6cm×5.3cm×5.4cm，盆腔前方有肿瘤 10.3cm×12.3cm×11.3cm，后方一个为 4.8cm×8.5cm×5.8cm，髂窝部左侧肿瘤 4.8cm×3.1cm×3.2cm，靠右侧肿瘤为 1.9cm×2cm×2.7cm 等。

腹部除了有这样多肿瘤还有大量腹水。肺部的情况也很差，右肺不张、实变并且还有胸腔积液，双下肢也严重水肿。腹腔大量肿瘤的压迫使得腹腔内脏器组织受压移位，这种病情是非常严重的。一个肿瘤的治疗就已经很困难了，这样多的大肿瘤，又伴有多脏器转移、腹水、胸腔积液、疼痛严重，为了活命，只能设法抽水。然而放腹水后第二天就又产生大量腹水，再加上很多的大肿瘤，患者的腹部已经无法承受，像是充气过多的气球，随时都会爆炸。医院明确表示已无法治疗，患者的痛苦可想而知。

因为疾病实在太严重，在万般无奈的情况下，2012 年 7 月 16 日汤女士的丈夫用轮椅推她到诊所中心求于生命修复抗癌症中医药治疗。

治则：扶正攻邪，排毒化瘀。

常用中药：黄芪、人参、牵牛子、红花、甘遂、大戟、芫花、芦荟、茯苓、水蛭、贝母、山慈菇。消瘤 1 号同时服用。

黄芪、茯苓、人参扶正利水，牵牛子、甘遂、大戟等均峻下逐水排毒，以遏止迅速增长的腹水、胸腔积液等，红花、水蛭等化瘀通经，加贝母、山慈菇等散结，起到消除肿瘤、攻逐水饮、扶正抗癌等功效。

其后继续用了中医药祛水、消瘤、散结、补正等不同治法，病情紧急及严重的程度逐渐缓解。之后她的腹部渐渐减小，精神状态也渐渐好转。治疗四个月后，肿瘤、腹水均明显减少，腹部外观恢复正常。汤女士也没有再去医院抽过水。

至 2015 年，患者已可以工作，后去国外，失访。

卵巢癌占女性生殖系统癌瘤的 20% 左右，卵巢癌的癌瘤位于腹腔深部，生长隐蔽，早期难以发现。如汤女士到肿瘤非常严重时才知道患了癌症。卵巢癌生长容易侵犯其他组织和脏器、破坏功能、压迫器官产生疼痛等各种症状，并容易发生腹腔种植和转移，这样严重的病况，目前尚没有公认的切实有效的常规治疗方法。但是，依靠医师对肿瘤深入的攻关研究和丰富的治疗经验，终于将不可治变为可治。

抗癌治验录 **下篇**

诊疗记录

2012年7月30日汤女士初来求诊时，腹内有大量肿瘤和腹水。

2012年10月，汤女士经治疗后，已恢复正常。

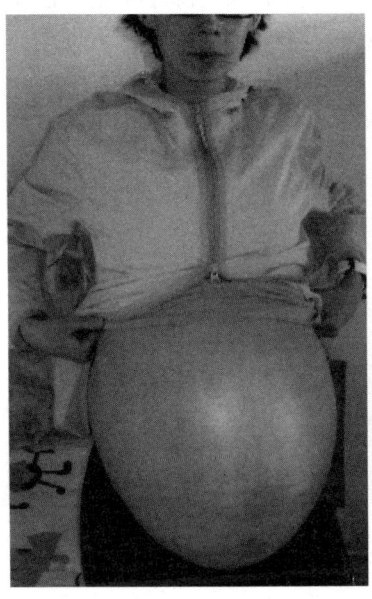

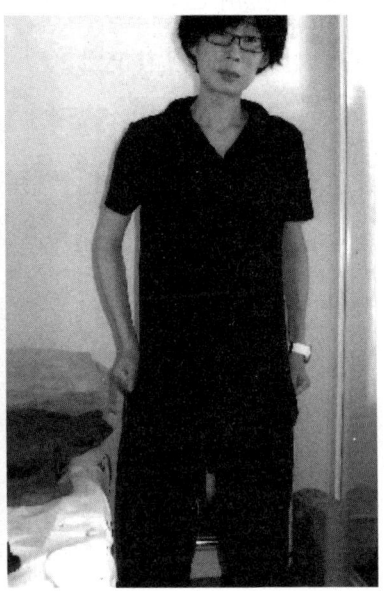

病案 22
停化疗扶阳祛毒，晚期肿瘤全消失

雷小姐（五十八岁）患直肠与结肠腺癌，2010年9月首次要求用抗癌中医药治疗。她在西医安排肿瘤切除手术前，已发现有大量癌细胞转移淋巴。

2010年9月她进行手术切除了五厘米大的肿瘤，术后病理报告证实为肠腺癌及淋巴转移。病理学诊断为：T3N2b期，即第三期淋巴转移。术后她按西医要求尽快接受了化疗，然而在此期间出现了严重不良反应，包括呕吐、全身疼痛、反胃及脸部水肿等。

化疗放疗饱受痛苦

雷小姐在进行化疗的同时前来寻求抗癌中医药治疗。当时主要是因为化疗的不良反应太大，她认为加用中医药调理，反应会减轻，使得化疗不那么痛苦。当然她还是觉得应以化疗为主要治疗手段。在化疗过程中，她经常出现呕吐、全身疼痛等症状，以后又发生脱发、腹泻、肝功能受损，也发生过严重的过敏反应，借中医药调理身体后，她的肝脏功能逐渐提升，化疗所带来不良作用减轻。

终于熬到六次化疗全部完成，又继续使用标靶药，医生之后还安排了二十八次放疗，在此期间她再一次出现腹痛、食不下咽、大量便血及腹泻等反应，但最后还是坚持完成了放疗。2011年2月完成放疗后，大便更是大量出血，血压也降低到正常值以下。放疗期间她采用中药辅助治疗，放疗后体内的肿瘤并没缩小。

西医又安排了新的化疗，雷小姐又咬牙坚持了下来，她唯一的希望是坚持完成这些化疗后，肿瘤就会消失，但在完成化疗后再检查，发现腹腔仍有多个肿瘤及多量淋巴转移。因腹腔肿瘤增大压迫到右腿阻碍了血液循环和回流，她自大腿以下全肢出现了严重水肿。CT检查结果显示有部分肿瘤缩小，但有更多肿瘤却增大，没有达到预期的效果，很多肿瘤仍然存在。

西医建议继续化疗，但雷小姐感到身体再也无法承受，于是决定不再接受化疗等西医治疗，专心用生命修复抗癌中医药治疗。

来诊时症见面色苍白、四肢无力、头晕耳鸣、恶心呕吐、便溏、便血、四肢无力，舌暗有瘀斑，脉细。

治则：健运中焦，益气养血。

常用中药：地榆、槐角、马齿苋、茜草、桃仁、莪术、三棱、川大黄、茯苓、山药、薏苡仁、苍术。消瘤粉同时服用。

患者湿盛阳亏，中气虚败，气滞血瘀，癌毒势盛，治疗当补正攻邪，益气养血，畅达气机，消灭肿瘤。地榆、槐角、马齿苋、茜草等凉血止血、解毒抗癌；三棱、莪术、川大黄、桃仁化瘀消滞攻积；茯苓、山药、薏苡仁、苍术健运中焦、祛湿益气。

在接受化疗与放疗期间，中医药曾帮助她舒缓了严重的毒副作用，停止化疗后，她决定将抗癌中药的力度加大。经过一段时间后，她已没有任何不适，下肢严重肿胀已渐减退消失，身体逐渐康复。

又过了几个月，雷小姐感觉良好。她就打算回医院详细检查身体，但因当时已没接受化疗或放疗，医院拒绝提供免费检查。因为当时身体状况良好，就决定尽量减少放射性检查的危害和减少费用，继续用抗癌中医药治疗，全凭中医的诊疗方法（望、闻、问、切）及全部天然植物进行治疗，而不做CT等检查。如果肿瘤有变化会出现临床表现和相应的症状，可以通过医生的基本功检查出来，不一定要通过有一定危害性的仪器检查才知道。就这样又继续服用中药一至两个月后，雷小姐还是没忍住，自行到私家医院做了检查，看看身体状况到底如何。

益气养血，攻毒补正

2012年8月，医院报告显示，她的所有肿瘤全部消失，转移的淋巴结包括腹腔、腹股沟、腹膜后的淋巴都全部消失。结果显示身体没有任何异常，健康正常。雷小姐在化疗期间，仍出现很多毒副作用，例如白细胞降低、呕吐、腹泻、脱发、疲累、肝功能异常、抽筋等，因此使用中药的原则为益气养血、解毒、补肝肾等。后来放疗期间出现便血、呕吐、腹泻、咽痛、失眠等，治疗则以益气养血，解毒止血为主，其后则以攻毒补正、排毒消瘤为主。至2017年，雷小姐患癌已有七年，每年检查都显示肿瘤无复发。这个成功的案例再一次说明：中医药可以治疗晚期肿瘤。

诊疗记录

2010年9月14日病理报告证实患肠腺癌淋巴血管浸润，大量淋巴转移。

2012年8月14日CT和PET检查报告证实肿瘤没有复发，淋巴转移病灶全部消失。

2013年5月23日再次检查，肿瘤全部消失，没有复发和转移。

治癌实录 2
中晚期癌症 · 名家手记

附：患者检查报告

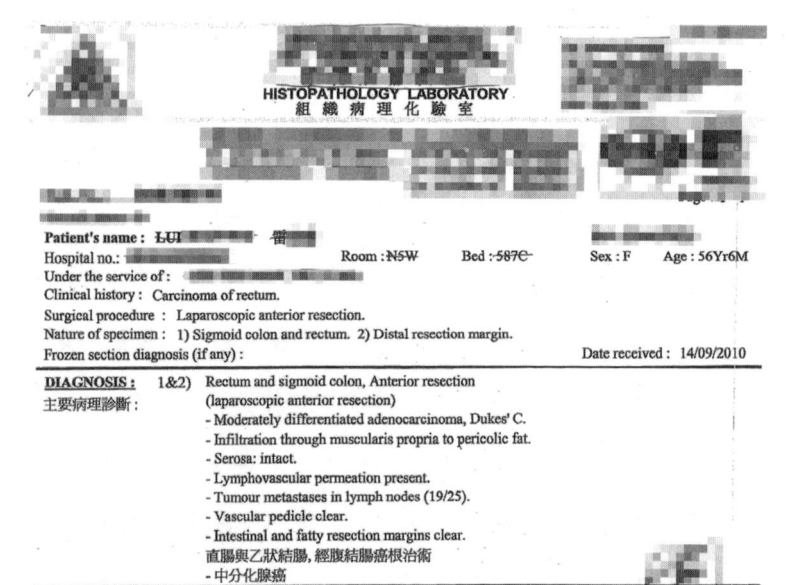

HISTOPATHOLOGY LABORATORY
組織病理化驗室

Patient's name: LUI ▓▓▓▓▓ 雷▓▓
Hospital no.: ▓▓▓▓▓▓▓▓ Room: NSW Bed: 587C Sex: F Age: 56Yr6M
Under the service of: ▓▓▓▓▓▓▓▓▓▓▓▓▓▓
Clinical history: Carcinoma of rectum.
Surgical procedure: Laparoscopic anterior resection.
Nature of specimen: 1) Sigmoid colon and rectum. 2) Distal resection margin.
Frozen section diagnosis (if any): Date received: 14/09/2010

DIAGNOSIS: 1&2) Rectum and sigmoid colon, Anterior resection
主要病理診斷： (laparoscopic anterior resection)
- Moderately differentiated adenocarcinoma, Dukes' C.
- Infiltration through muscularis propria to pericolic fat.
- Serosa: intact.
- Lymphovascular permeation present.
- Tumour metastases in lymph nodes (19/25).
- Vascular pedicle clear.
- Intestinal and fatty resection margins clear.
直腸與乙狀結腸，經腹結腸癌根治術
- 中分化腺癌

MACROSCOPIC EXAMINATION: Printed on: 15/09/2010 11:16:04

(KCH, mk)

1) Sigmoid and rectum. A segment of sigmoid colon including the rectum is submitted. It measures 13.5 cm long with a diameter of 2.6 cm. It has been cut opened upon submission. The anterior peritoneal reflection is located at 2.3 cm proximal to the distal resection margin. At the right posterolateral surface of the colon, there is an ulcerated tumour measuring 4.4 cm longitudinally. It is located at 3.4 cm from the distal resection margin and 6.7 cm from the proximal resection margin. The tumour occupies about 70% of the luminal area. The tumour is located at 1.1 cm above of the anterior peritoneal reflection. Cut surface of the tumour shows transmural tumour infiltration into the pericolic fatty tissue. The serosa is not infiltrated by tumour. There is no serosal nodule present. The tumour is far from the adventitial fat resection margin measuring about 3.9 cm away from it. There is no satellite tumour nodule present in the mucosa. At the mesentery, there is an area with fibrous induration. This focus measures 0.5 cm across. About 25 lymph nodes are sampled from the pericolic fatty tissue with some of them being matted in appearance. The largest one measures 2.8 cm across. The largest lymph node is focally close to the fatty resection margin. Tissue blocks are taken as follows: (A) Intestinal resection margins, 2 tissue blocks. Nearest adventival margin from the tumour, 1 tissue block. (B)to(E) Tumour, 4 tissue blocks. (F) The area of induration of the mesentery, 2 tissue blocks. (G) Apical vascular pedicle, 1 tissue block. (H)to(J) The smaller lymph nodes, multiple tissue blocks. (K)to(L) The largest lymph node, 2 representative blocks with inclusion of the adventitial resection margin which is dyed black. Figure 1 shows the submitted specimen. Figure 2 shows the close-up view of the tumour. Figure 3 shows cut surface of the tumour. Figure 4 shows the area of induration in the mesentery.

2) Distal resection margin. A ring of mucosa covered tissue measuring 2.5 x 2 cm with a thickness of 0.6 cm. All embedded.

to be continued ......

抗癌治验录 下篇

Name:	Lui,			Date:	14/08/2012
I.D. No.:		Sex:	Female	Ref. Dr.:	
Hosp. No.:		Age:	58 Y	Fax:	
Ward/Dept.:	Clinical Oncology	ExamID:		Tel:	

POSITRON EMISSION TOMOGRAPHY
(^{18}F-FDG ONCOLOGY)

History:

A 58 year-old lady had laparoscopic resection of upper rectum in 09/2010, T3N2b disease, followed by chemotherapy and radiation therapy. PET here in 03/2011 showed mildly active nodes along right iliac vessel, aortocaval and paracaval regions. After 1 more cycle of chemotherapy, it was stopped due to side-effects. She switched to herbal medicine but later complained of right lower limb swelling. PET in 6/2011 showed improvement of myositis and nodes. She continued with herbal medicine, but sustained a recent minor trauma to her lower right chest wall. Hysterectomy for fibroid, cholecystectomy and appendectomy.

Radiopharmaceutical: 10.9 mCi F-18 Fluorodeoxyglucose (^{18}FDG) injected intravenously.

Findings:

Limited whole body CT transmission and PET emission imaging began at 84 minutes after radiopharmaceutical administration (blood glucose 5.4 mmol/l), spanning a region from base of skull to upper thigh. 60 mg Spasmonal was given p.o. 15 min before ^{18}FDG administration.

Liver tissue normal reference uptake has a SUVmax of 2.53.

The current examination is compared with prior study of 06/2011. The rectal anastomosis is marked by radiopaque sutures. It shows no metabolic evidence of local tumor recurrence. The anastomotic bowel loops show normal activities. The hypermetabolic lymph nodes previously observed in the right pelvic cavity, right groin and retroperitoneum have completely resolved. No evidence of hypermetabolic lymphadenopathy detected during this evaluation. There is still mildly increased gluteal muscle activity just adjacent to right hip joint, consistent with mild inflammatory activities, bilateral involving both sides. Physiologic bowel activities are noted in the ascending and transverse colon. There is no interval lymphadenopathy within the mesentery or omentum. The liver, adrenal glands, pancreas and spleen show normal size and metabolism. Kidney configuration is normal.

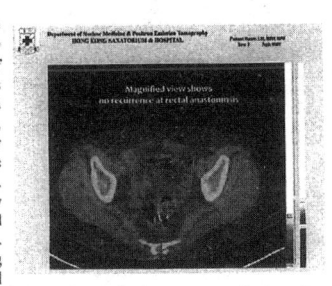

In the thorax, there remains normal parenchymal and pleural activity of bilateral lung segments. The tiny nodule in the inferolateral LUL is still ~2-3 mm, stable and without abnormal metabolism. No pleural or pericardial effusion. There is no lymphadenopathy in bilateral hila, mediastinum, supraclavicular fossae or jugular lymphatics.

Skeletal survey shows no abnormal marrow metabolism. Specially, there is no abnormal activity involving the right lower chest cage to suggest the presence of metabolically active pathology.
Functional parameters to compare these 2 studies are tabulated below:

Lui,	Current Study Date 14.08.2012 in mm				Current Study Date 15.06.2011 in mm				SUVmax% change
Site	LD	PD	SUVmax	TLG	LD	PD	SUVmax	TLG	
Rt gluteal muscle	-	-	3.0	-	-	-	3.4	-	-12.1%

Note: LD=longest diameter; PD=diameter perpendicular to LD; TLG=total lesion glycolysis (vol x SUVmean)

Impression:

1. No PET/CT evidence of local recurrence or regional metastatic lymphadenopathy given patient's history of treatment for rectal malignancy.
2. All the previously detected hypermetabolic pelvic, groin and retroperitoneal nodes have metabolically and physically resolved.
3. Mild residual gluteal muscle activities adjacent to bilateral hips suggest mild myositis.
4. Stable 2-3 mm lung nodule in the LUL, likely benign.
5. No evidence of interval distant metastasis.

Thank you very much, for your referral.

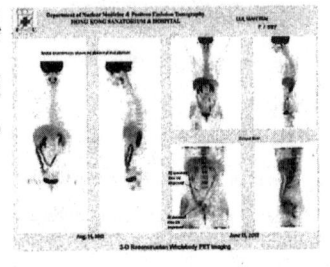

MD(HK), MBBS(HK), MSc(Stanford), ABNM,CBNC
Department of Nuclear Medicine & P.E.T., HKSH

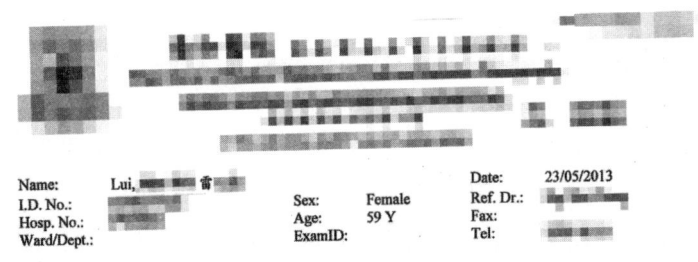

Name:	Lui,	Sex:	Female	Date:	23/05/2013
I.D. No.:		Age:	59 Y	Ref. Dr.:	
Hosp. No.:		ExamID:		Fax:	
Ward/Dept.:				Tel:	

POSITRON EMISSION TOMOGRAPHY
(^{18}F-FDG ONCOLOGY)

History:

A 59 year-old lady had laparoscopic resection of upper rectum in 09/2010, T3N2b disease, followed by chemotherapy and radiation therapy. PET here in 03/2011 showed mildly active nodes along right iliac vessel, aortocaval and paracaval regions. After 1 more cycle of chemotherapy, it was stopped due to side-effects. She switched to herbal medicine but later complained of right lower limb swelling. PET in 6/2011 showed improvement of myositis and nodes. She continued with herbal medicine. PET scan in 08/2012 showed no evidence of disease recurrence. Clinically asymptomatic. No further treatment was given. Hysterectomy for fibroid, cholecystectomy and appendectomy. Tumor marker found not useful for monitoring.

Radiopharmaceutical: 9.8 mCi F-18 Fluorodeoxyglucose (^{18}FDG) injected intravenously.

Findings:

Limited whole body CT transmission and PET emission imaging began at 60 minutes after radiopharmaceutical administration (blood glucose 5.2 mmol/l), spanning a region from base of skull to upper thigh. 60 mg Spasmonal was given p.o. 15 min before ^{18}FDG administration.

Liver tissue normal reference uptake has a SUVmax of 2.95.

Comparison is made with the prior study performed here in 08/2012. Patient is status post laparoscopic resection of rectal malignancy and radiation therapy. Surgery of the entire colon including the rectal suture shows no metabolic evidence of local recurrent disease. There is no hypermetabolic lymphadenopathy in bilateral groins, ischiorectal fossae, along iliac vessels or great vessels in the abdomen. The metastatic nodes in the retoperitoneum have subsided for 2 consecutive scans, in keeping with metabolic remission. No abnormal focal glycolysis in the omentum, mesentery, presacral regions and pelvic sidewall. There is no ascites.

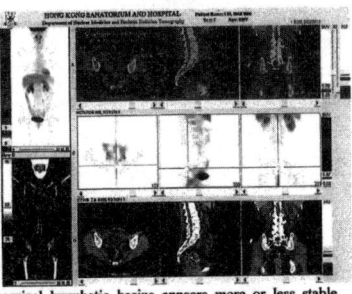

The small mildly active node in right upper cervical lymphatic basins appears more or less stable, suggestive of reactive node. Physiologic nasopharyngeal and thyroidal activity is present. In the thorax, there is normal parenchymal and pleural activity. The tiny nodule in inferolateral LUL remains stable and non active, suggestive of old granuloma. No hypermetabolic lymphadenopathy in bilateral hila and mediastinum. No pleural effusion. Bilateral axillae and breasts appear unremarkable. In the abdomen, there is normal size and metabolism in liver, spleen, adrenal glands and pancreas. No abnormal focal glycolysis in the stomach or the hysterectomy bed. Skeletal survey shows no hypermetabolic marrow activity to suggest active osseous metastasis. The myositis activities around bilateral hips are barely visible.

Impression:

1. No PET/CT evidence of local recurrence or regional metastatic lymphadenopathy given patient's history of treatment for rectal malignancy.
2. The hypermetabolic retroperitoneal nodes have subsided for 2 consecutive scans, in keeping with metabolic remission.
3. Stable reactive right upper cervical node and LUL tiny nodule.
4. No evidence of distant metastasis.
5. In summery: clinical remission.

Thank you very much, ▇▇▇, for your referral.

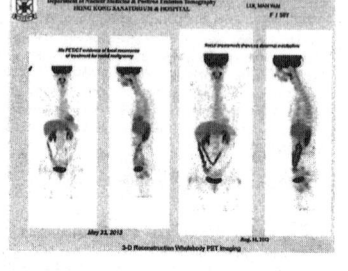

, MBChB, MSc (Lond), FHKCR, FHKAM (Radiology)
Specialist in Nuclear Medicine, Department of Nuclear Medicine & P.E.T., HKSH

病案 23
咳喘原从腮腺来，清热解毒助瘤消

2006年陈先生在50岁的时候，因咳嗽、气喘去医院就诊。他多次服用医生开的治咳药水后，咳嗽、气喘仍旧不见好转，且因此拖延数月而致病情加重，后来做肺部的进一步检查，发现两肺有多发性肿瘤。陈先生和家人得知消息后非常悲伤难过，感到生命不久了，心情也变得烦躁不安、失眠、抑郁，进一步检查发现，情况更加糟糕，其所患的癌症已到晚期，双肺的多发肿瘤并不是原发的，而是身体其他部位转移来的。又经过全身的多次检查、抽取组织做病理学检查等，最后证实为原发于腮腺的癌症，已经侵犯到面神经、双肺等多处。

陈先生曾接受了西医的放疗，又做了一次化疗，之后感到身体不能承受，咳嗽气喘都加重，而且出现了呼吸困难、不能平卧等严重症状。之后西医检查发现CT报告显示两侧肺部肿瘤大量增多，密密麻麻，一侧的肺上至少有50处，两肺至少有100处，所以只能放弃化疗，在走投无路的情况下，陈先生和太太一起来到了我们的诊所。

陈先生来诊时，面色暗黑、十分消瘦、气短不续、呼吸困难、咳嗽不止、血痰、声嘶、因为肿瘤压迫而致右侧面瘫、头痛难忍、眼睑下垂不能睁开、口眼㖞斜、口水下流，而且在他的右侧耳部也有一个转移的肿瘤，占据了整个耳廓，耳道及耳孔被严严实实地堵住，造成其听力的严重障碍，右侧耳完全不能听到声音。舌红少苔，脉细数。

治则： 清热解毒、攻坚消瘤。

常用中药： 天花粉、草河车、夏枯草、半夏、黄药子、石上柏、山豆根、露蜂房、天葵子、贝母、猫抓草。散结粉同时服用。

天花粉、草河车，甘寒，清热解毒；夏枯草、半夏、黄药子、石上柏、山豆根、露蜂房、天葵子、贝母、猫爪草，清热解毒，散结消瘤。夏枯草苦寒，清热解郁散结，得至阳之气而长，半夏温燥，消痞散结，得至阴之气而生，二药寒温并用，相辅相成，加强散结功效。

本方大多数药味，均具解毒、攻坚散结之功效，并具有现代医学研究之抗癌作用，联合运用力量更强，终于消除了陈先生双肺的 100 处肿瘤结节。

2016 年 6 月随访时，陈先生生活愉快，工作紧张，在一家工厂负责技术工作。